Living with
Diabetes

Living with Diabetes

The Diabetes UK Guide for those Treated with Insulin

New Edition

Dr John L. Day
The Ipswich Hospital, UK

JOHN WILEY & SONS, LTD

Chichester • New York • Weinheim • Brisbane • Singapore • Toronto

First published 1998 by John Wiley & Sons Ltd, Baffins Lane, Chichester, West Sussex
PO19 1UD, England
New Edition published 2002
   National   01243 779777   International (+44) 1243 779777
   e-mail (for orders and customer service enquiries): cs-books@wiley.co.uk
   Visit our Home Page on http://www.wiley.co.uk or http://www.wiley.com

Other Wiley Editorial Offices

John Wiley & Sons, Inc., 605 Third Avenue, New York, NY 10158-0012, USA

WILEY-VCH Verlag GmbH, Pappelallee 3, D-69469 Weinheim, Germany

Jacaranda Wiley Ltd, 33 Park Road, Milton, Queensland 4064, Australia

John Wiley & Sons (Asia) Pte Ltd, 2 Clementi Loop #02-01, Jin Xing Distripark, Singapore 129809

John Wiley & Sons (Canada) Ltd, 22 Worcester Road, Rexdale, Ontario M9W 1L1, Canada

British Library Cataloguing in Publication Data

A catalogue record for this book is available from the British Library

ISBN 0-470-84526-0

Typeset in 11/13 pt Plantin from the author's disks by
Hilite Design & Reprographics Ltd, Southampton, Hampshire
· Graphical illustrations by Ann Postill Technical Tracing & Allied Services, Guildford, Surrey;
Medical illustrations by Peter Lamb, Lambda Science Artwork, Corfu, Greece; Cartoons by
Clinton Banbury, Illustration & Design, Billericay, Essex
Printed and bound in Great Britain by L & S Printing Company Ltd, Worthing, West Sussex
This book is printed on acid-free paper responsibly manufactured from sustainable forestry, in
which at least two trees are planted for each one used for paper production.

Contents

Acknowledgements

I wish to acknowledge the important contributions to this book from J Rowley BSc SRD, Dietitian, A Blain SRN, and Claire Wadham of the Ipswich Diabetes Centre and, in particular, E Bartlett (Diabetes UK) who has been responsible for many of the amendments in this edition.

The Balance of Good Health Plate on page 52 is reproduced with kind permission of the Food Standards Agency, Aviation House, 125 Kingsway, London WC2B 6NH.

'A lot' and 'A little' figures on page 63 reproduced by permission of MAFF (now Department for Environment, Food & Rural Affairs) from Foodsense booklet *Use Your Label* (PB2362 – © Crown copyright).

The self-check height and weight chart on page 66 is reprinted from *Treat Obesity Seriously*, J. S Garrow, 1981, by permission of the publisher Churchill Livingstone, with acknowledgement to The Health Education Council, E Fullard, Oxford, and Servier Laboratories Limited, UK.

The illustration of the Active Erection Assistance System on page 132 was kindly supplied by Genesis Medical (Sales) Limited, Linton House, 39–51 Highgate Road, London NW5 1RT, and is reproduced here by their kind permission.

The illustration of a school dining hall on page 165 was kindly supplied by Headcorn County Primary School, Kings Road, Headcorn, Kent.

The illustrations of the scout on page 172, the adolescent party on page 179, the family meal on page 183 and the adolescent disco on page 203 were kindly supplied by Edward Hannan, Trumpeter, Water Lane, Headcorn, Kent.

1 Introducing Diabetes

■ About diabetes

The purpose of this book

Diabetes or, to give it its full name, diabetes mellitus, is very common. In the United Kingdom there are 1.4 million people known to have diabetes, of whom 20 000 are aged under 20. Diabetes UK believes that there may be as many as another 1 million people who remain undiagnosed. Worldwide there are over 151 million cases.

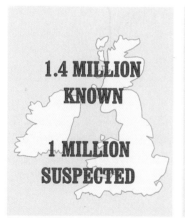 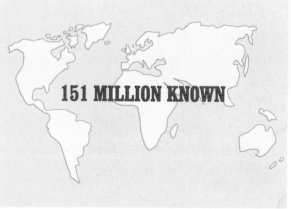

The estimated numbers of people with diabetes

Diabetes cannot be cured. However, you will see that there are steps you can take to ensure that the effects on your life are kept to a minimum.

You may wish to know more about the causes of diabetes to avoid undue worry that it is your own, or somebody else's, fault.

The aim of this book is to encourage you: to follow the recommended treatment with optimism; to share your concerns with those available to help; to be able to discuss your diabetes and its effects freely and without embarrassment with your friends, relatives, colleagues; and to attend regularly for the medical checks that are necessary from time to time.

If you are reading this book, either you have discovered that you have diabetes, or you are finding out more to help a relative or friend. You are not expected to read the book from cover to cover, but you may wish just to check on certain details or to refresh your memory on some aspects. The chapters have been divided with these possibilities in mind.

What is diabetes?

Diabetes is a disorder in which the mechanism for converting glucose to energy no longer functions properly. This causes an abnormally high level of glucose in the blood, giving rise to a variety of symptoms. If the glucose levels remain high over several years, damage may be caused to various parts of the body. Treatment of diabetes is designed not only to reverse symptoms but also to prevent any serious problems developing later.

How does diabetes develop?

Normally, the amount of glucose in the body is very carefully controlled. We obtain glucose from the food we eat, either from sweet things or from starchy foods (carbohydrates), such as bread and potatoes. Glucose can also be made by breaking down the body stores of starch in the liver. This will occur when the body needs an extra supply of glucose. This happens if you miss several meals, or have been injured, or are unwell.

The use of glucose to provide energy requires the presence of the chemical hormone, insulin. Insulin is released into the blood as the blood glucose rises after a meal. Its function is to return the glucose concentration to its original level. Less insulin is produced when the glucose level falls, for example during exercise. Insulin plays a vital role in maintaining the correct level of blood glucose.

When there is a shortage of insulin, or if the available insulin does not function correctly, then the blood glucose rises and diabetes results.

The blood glucose level of someone who does not have diabetes normally varies between 3.5 and 9.0 mmol/l.

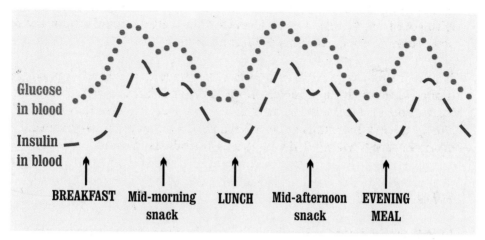

Insulin rising and falling in response to the blood glucose. This shows the blood glucose rising after each meal or snack. This rise stimulates the release of insulin. The insulin returns the glucose level to normal

A little history

Diabetes cannot be called a 'modern' condition. It was referred to in ancient Egyptian, Indian, Roman, Japanese and Chinese writings.

However, no significant advance was made in understanding the nature of diabetes until the 19th century. The first major breakthrough came in 1889. Two German scientists discovered that the removal of the pancreas, a large gland in the abdomen, gave rise to diabetes. It was also discovered that damage to clusters of cells in the pancreas, called islets of Langerhans, produced certain forms of diabetes. It was not until 1921 that two Canadians, Frederick Banting and Charles Best, made their famous discovery of insulin.

Who gets diabetes? Why?

In the United Kingdom, as many as three people in every 100 have diabetes, and perhaps one in every 600 schoolchildren. It can occur at any age, but is very rare in infants. It is more common in people approaching middle-age and in older people.

There are two main types of diabetes.

■ Type 1 – Insulin dependent diabetes.

■ Type 2 – Non insulin dependent diabetes.

Type 1 – Insulin dependent diabetes

Cause

In this type of diabetes there is a complete absence of insulin, due to the destruction of the insulin-producing cells. With this type of diabetes it is essential to have insulin treatment to survive.

The exact cause of the damage to the insulin-producing cells is not known for certain, but a combination of factors may be involved including:

■ Damage to the insulin-producing cells by viral or other infections
■ An abnormal reaction of the body against the insulin-producing cells.

Who gets it?

In general, Type 1 diabetes is first diagnosed in younger people (under 40 years of age), but occasionally it occurs in older people, even the very old. Both sexes are equally affected.

There is some tendency for this type of diabetes to run in families, but the condition is far from being entirely inherited.

Type 2 – Non insulin dependent diabetes

Cause

If you have Type 2 (non insulin dependent) diabetes you are still producing insulin, but it is either not being made in sufficient quantities or not working properly. You do not need to take insulin in order to survive. Most people with Type 2 diabetes can be treated effectively by diet and exercise, or by a combination of diet and tablets. Sometimes insulin injections may be necessary to establish good control of blood glucose levels. If you do require insulin it doesn't mean that you have developed Type 1 diabetes. It just means that you need a little more help to keep your Type 2 diabetes under control. Despite continuing research the cause is not yet known.

Who gets it?

Type 2 diabetes used to be called 'maturity onset diabetes'. This was because it occurs mainly in the middle and older age groups, although it can sometimes occur in younger people. Overweight people are particularly likely to develop this type of diabetes. People from African-Caribbean and Asian backgrounds are more commonly affected. It tends to run in families.

Other causes of diabetes

Diseases of the pancreas

A very few cases of diabetes are due to various diseases of the pancreas. These include inflammation (pancreatitis) or unusual deposits of iron. Mumps may sometimes have the same effect.

Accidents or illness

Major accidents or illnesses do not cause diabetes. However, they do sometimes produce a temporary increase in blood glucose.

If your diabetes was discovered during the course of an illness, it is most likely that you already had diabetes (even though you may not have had any symptoms). Some forms of hormone imbalance may also produce temporary diabetes.

Tablets

Some tablets can increase the blood glucose and reveal pre-existing diabetes. Steroid drugs or water tablets which eliminate fluid from the body (diuretics) may do this.

The contraceptive pill

This does not cause diabetes, but it may raise the blood glucose slightly.

Heredity

If one parent has diabetes, his or her children are slightly more likely than average to develop diabetes. The risk, however, is small. For example, the chances of developing diabetes before the age of 20 are perhaps only one in 100. Rarely, both parents have diabetes, in which case the chances are increased.

Type 2 (non insulin dependent) diabetes is more commonly inherited than Type 1 (insulin dependent) diabetes. However, this form usually occurs in people who are middle-aged or older, therefore their children are not usually affected until later in life. This is more likely to happen if such children become overweight when they are middle-aged, although it is increasingly being seen in younger people.

To summarise, it is possible for someone to inherit a tendency to diabetes, but not to inherit the condition itself. This only develops because of some other influence. Thus, there are very many people with a strong family history of the disorder who never develop diabetes.

Onset of symptoms and their severity

The main symptoms of diabetes are:

- Increased thirst and a dry mouth
- Passing frequent amounts of urine especially at night
- Weight loss
- Extreme tiredness
- Itching of the genital organs
- Blurring of vision.

Symptoms vary considerably in their severity and rate of onset, but they can all be rapidly relieved by treatment.

Type 1 (insulin dependent) diabetes

The symptoms develop fairly quickly, usually over a few weeks. Sometimes they come on quite quickly over just a few days. Without insulin treatment the condition progressively worsens, resulting in a significant weight loss, dehydration, vomiting, the onset of drowsiness and diabetic coma.

Type 2 (non insulin dependent) diabetes

The symptoms are similar to those of Type 1 diabetes, but they develop more gradually and are usually less severe. Diabetic coma does not occur in this type of diabetes.

Some people with diabetes fail to notice any symptoms, but after being treated they usually have more energy and feel considerably better. Unfortunately, the presence of symptoms is no guide to the level of glucose in the blood, and it is essential that diabetes is treated, even when there are no symptoms.

Treatment

Diabetes is a very common disorder. Although no 'cure' is yet possible, all types of diabetes can be treated and normal health restored.

Treatment is with:

■ Insulin and diet – for
Type 1 (insulin dependent)
diabetes

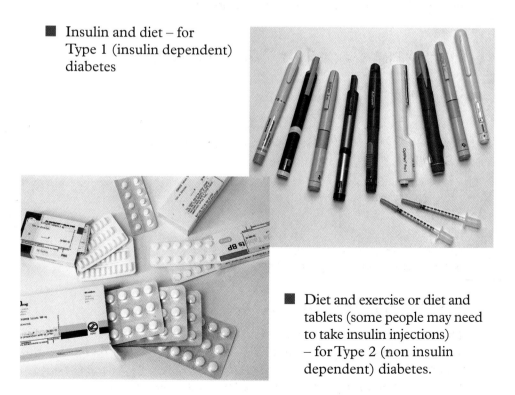

■ Diet and exercise or diet and
tablets (some people may need
to take insulin injections)
– for Type 2 (non insulin
dependent) diabetes.

Treatment must be maintained throughout life. This is necessary not only to avoid symptoms and the risk of coma, but also to minimise the risks of any later complications.

All forms of treatment require some modification to daily routines, and the performance of checks to ensure that treatment is effective. However, you should be able to achieve these with only minimal disturbance to your daily life.

From Chapter 2 onwards, this book explains in detail what has gone wrong in your type of diabetes. You will see how, with correct treatment, you should be able to maintain effective control.

Modern treatment allows the many thousands of people with diabetes to achieve complete, fruitful, healthy lives. Diabetes should not interfere with the vast majority of occupations. Many of the most successful people in the country not only have diabetes, but have fulfilled their ambitions in all walks of life. These include first-class sportsmen and women, politicians, actors, actresses, and successful members of all professions, people who bear witness to the fact that effective treatment can be combined with the highest achievement.

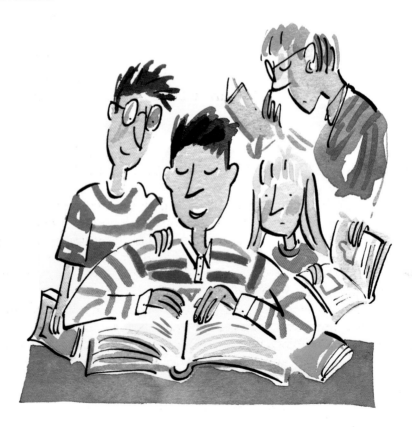

2 Type 1 (Insulin Dependent) Diabetes

When your diabetes was diagnosed, you will have been told that you need to have regular insulin injections. These are essential for you to return to and maintain good health. The objectives of this chapter are to explain:

- How insulin controls glucose in the body.
- What has happened in your case.
- Why it may have occurred.
- The reasons for any symptoms you may have experienced.
- Why treatment is necessary even if you have had no symptoms.
- Why treatment must be continued.

■ Normal glucose control in the body

In Chapter 1 the role of glucose control in the development of diabetes was briefly considered. To understand this further you need to know some facts about the food you eat. This is made up of three basic types – carbohydrates, fats and proteins. These three types of food are broken down by digestive processes in the intestine. The products are then absorbed into the blood stream and carried to the individual body cells. Carbohydrates, found in starchy foods such as bread and potatoes, are broken down and converted to glucose. Fat is converted to fatty acids. Fatty acids and glucose are used to provide energy in the body. When protein is digested amino acids are produced. These are used to build cells and tissues. Any excess is converted to glucose.

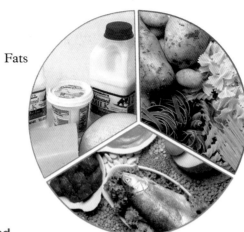

Fats

Carbohydrates
(starches
and sugars)

**Fats, carbohydrates and
proteins are essential**

Proteins

All three types of food are essential (see opposite). The majority of energy is provided by glucose. The diet must therefore contain sufficient carbohydrate. Some fat and protein is necessary to ensure that the body cells have a supply of the nutrients they require.

Where does blood glucose come from?

In the healthy individual, the level of blood glucose is kept within close limits. The major source of glucose is the food we eat. Blood glucose therefore goes up after a meal. It normally reaches a peak about 60–90 minutes after eating. Then as time passes the level falls again. The main sources of blood glucose in food are:

- ◼ Sweet things, eg extra sugar added to cereals, sugary drinks, jams, etc
- ◼ Starchy foods, eg bread, potatoes, rice, pasta, cereals, chapattis, cassava, yam, etc
- ◼ Other foods, eg protein may be converted to glucose.

When our food intake provides more glucose than the body needs at the time, the excess is stored in the liver. This store acts as a reserve for times of need, illness or injury. Once the liver stores are filled, any excess is converted to fat. This is what happens if you eat too much over a long period. Too much of the other fuels (fats and proteins) will ultimately have the same effect – both blood glucose and body weight will increase.

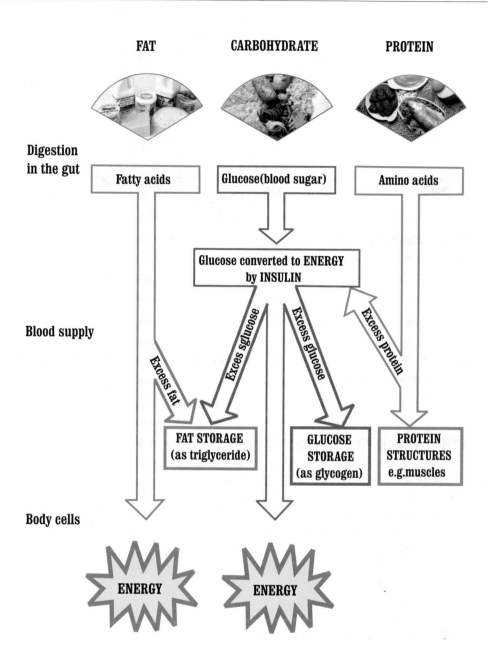

Normal metabolism. In the presence of insulin, glucose can be converted to energy

The importance of insulin

Insulin is the key to the conversion of glucose to energy (or its storage). It also helps to maintain the amount of stored energy by stopping excessive breakdown of fat. Insulin is produced by the pancreas. This is a gland situated at the back of the abdomen. As can be seen in the diagram below, this gland contains little groups of cells, called the islets of Langerhans. These cells sense the level of glucose in the blood. They then send just the right amount of insulin into the blood to dispose of it.

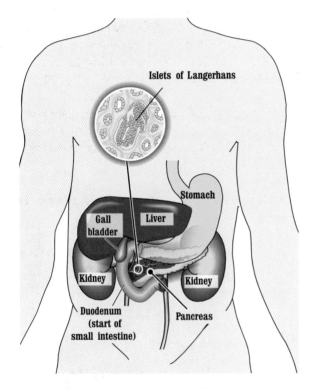

The pancreas. The pancreas is a large gland positioned behind the stomach. It contains many cells which produce insulin. These occur in clusters called islets of Langerhans

What has gone wrong?

In your type of diabetes these insulin-producing cells have been damaged so that your pancreas either produces insufficient insulin or none at all. It is thus not possible to convert the glucose from the diet into energy or to store it effectively. In the absence of insulin, fat is broken down. Fat breakdown products build up in the blood. Weight is lost. This is what happens in Type 1 (insulin dependent) diabetes, and why it is necessary to inject insulin regularly in order to control the blood glucose level.

Why has this happened?

The exact cause is uncertain. A virus probably caused the initial damage. The damaged cells release chemicals which start a chain reaction causing gradual loss of all the insulin-producing cells. This cannot, unfortunately, be reversed. The damage probably took place several years before your symptoms started. If everything else, however, is working normally, you can and will remain fit and well once the insulin is being replaced.

Although this type of diabetes is not strictly inherited you may have other family members with the same problem. You have probably inherited a tendency to develop diabetes, but this is not the major cause. Many people with this tendency never develop the disorder.

Type 1 (insulin dependent) diabetes usually affects young people, but it may occur in middle and later years.

Always remember that your diabetes has not been caused by eating the wrong things. In particular, sugar itself does not cause diabetes.

How does insulin work?

Whenever we eat, the blood glucose level rises. This is the signal for insulin to go into action. Normally, insulin pours out of the pancreas during the half hour after a meal. This insulin is responsible for reducing the blood glucose level.

The graph on the next page (above) shows the blood glucose rising after a meal. As soon as the glucose level begins to rise, the pancreas detects the change and immediately starts releasing insulin into the blood, as shown in the graph on the next page (below). As the insulin speeds through the circulation, it allows glucose to penetrate into the body cells, so that about two hours after a meal, the blood glucose falls back to the pre-meal level.

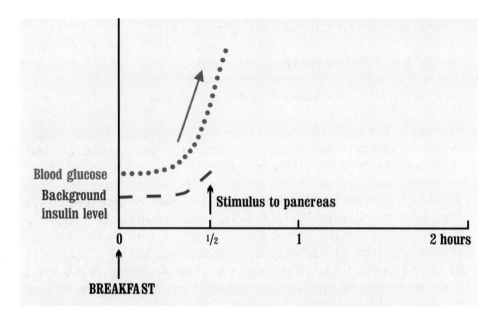

Blood glucose rising during the half hour after a meal

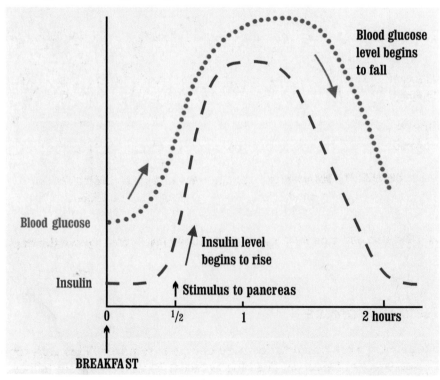

Insulin released from the pancreas makes the blood glucose level fall

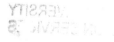

Thus, there are two important facts to remember:

1. The blood glucose rises after each meal.

2. Insulin brings the glucose level down to normal.

Whenever we eat, the blood glucose rises and it is at this time, therefore, that we need an extra boost of insulin to convert the glucose to energy, and thus make it available for use by the body cells.

Insulin production keeps very closely in step with glucose levels, as can be seen from the diagram below. It is important to appreciate that these are extra boosts of insulin. Between meals there is always a steady background release of insulin. This is because between meals there is a steady trickle of glucose from the liver, which stops the blood glucose from falling too low when we are not eating. The slow release of insulin ensures that this glucose is used, thus enabling the cells to keep 'ticking over'.

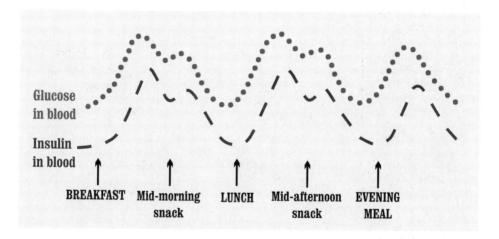

Insulin levels keep closely in step with glucose levels throughout the day

Effect of exercise

During heavy work or exercise, more energy is required. This calls for an increased supply of glucose. The blood glucose is prevented from falling too low by receiving a top-up from the liver. If, however, the insulin level should be too high, as can occur in those who inject insulin, the liver may not be able to keep up its supply of glucose. The blood glucose level falls too low. We call this state of low blood glucose hypoglycaemia (*hypo* = low, *gly* = glucose, *aemia* = in the blood). Exercise can cause hypoglycaemia. Thus, control of the blood glucose depends on a 'balance' between the supply of glucose from food or the liver and its disposal as energy or stored energy. This balance, which depends directly on the amount of insulin available and what you have eaten, is illustrated in the diagram below.

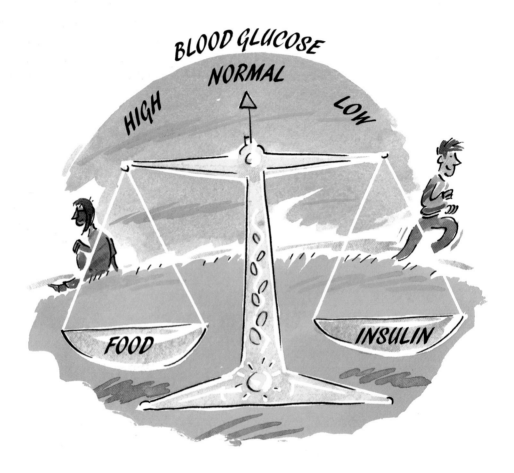

Control = Balance. Good control of blood glucose depends on a balance between the glucose from the diet and the amount of insulin produced. This balance can be altered by the effects of exercise, or lack of it

■ What happens without insulin?

The blood glucose rises

Without insulin the body is unable to use the glucose from the blood to obtain the energy it needs. After a meal, therefore, the blood glucose rises too high (hyperglycaemia). In addition, if glucose is not required to provide energy any excess is normally stored in the liver. This is then released slowly at times of need, for example if you go without eating for several hours, or overnight. Insulin controls this release. Without insulin this release continues uncontrollably and the blood glucose continues to rise even when you are not eating. This is made worse if the body needs are increased. This happens if you are ill or injured. When the system is working normally more insulin is released to control this.

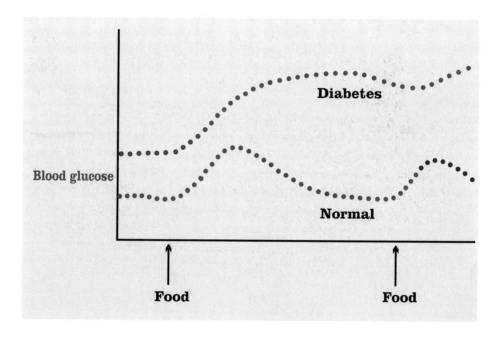

The effects of diabetes on blood glucose. In diabetes, insufficient insulin results in an excessively high blood glucose. It starts higher than normal and goes on rising after eating

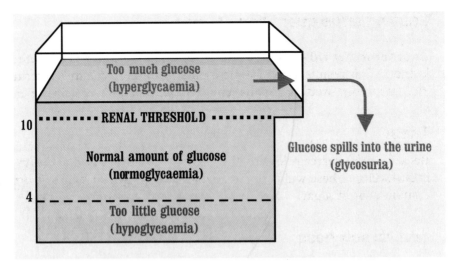

Blood glucose levels. When the blood glucose reaches a certain level it spills over into the urine. This level is called the renal threshold

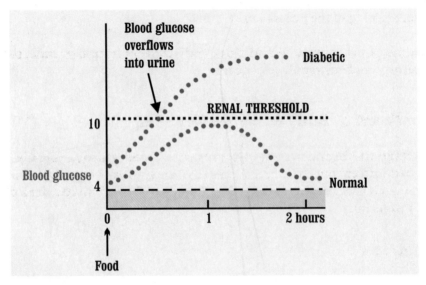

Glycosuria. The blood glucose rises above the renal threshold because of lack of insulin, and spills over into the urine

— *Glucose in the urine*

When there is too little insulin, however, the blood glucose reaches too high a level. It then starts to spill over into the urine in ever-increasing quantities. This is called glycosuria. Glycosuria gives rise to three of the commonest symptoms of uncontrolled diabetes:

Passing large quantities of urine

In order to get rid of the excess glucose, more water is excreted by the kidneys. This results in the frequent passing of large volumes of urine. It can give rise to bed-wetting in some children, and incontinence in the elderly.

Thirst

Because more water is leaving the body, a dry mouth and a feeling of thirst may develop. These will actually be made worse by drinking soft drinks that contain a lot of sugar.

Genital soreness

When large quantities of glucose are passed in the urine, it tends to create soreness around the genital area. It frequently causes itching of the vulva in women (in whom thrush is more likely to develop). Less frequently, it produces itching of the penis in men.

Once diabetes is controlled and glucose disappears from the urine, these unpleasant problems rapidly disappear.

Breakdown of body energy stores

A shortage or absence of insulin prevents blood glucose from being converted into energy. Therefore a source of energy must be provided from elsewhere. Consequently, there is a breakdown of fat and protein (muscle), which results in:

Weight loss

Diabetes is one of the commonest causes of weight loss, and occurs in most people at the onset of the disorder. It ranges from a few pounds to two or three stone in some of the more severe cases.

Tiredness and weakness

Tiredness, often accompanied by a sensation of weakness, is very common in uncontrolled diabetes. Some people are more than usually prone to fall asleep at odd times, while others just feel they are growing old before their time. This symptom can be completely reversed by treatment. Many feel 'rejuvenated' after starting treatment, even when they had previously been unaware of any abnormalities.

An increased appetite

In some individuals there is a noticeable increase in appetite.

Ketoacidosis

Ketoacidosis (also called ketosis or diabetic coma) is a complication of insulin deficiency which must be avoided at all costs. It is caused by a severe lack of insulin. This is particularly likely when the body's need for insulin is increased, such as during an infection or an illness.

If insulin is completely absent the liver, besides swamping the blood with glucose, tries to replace this fuel by breaking down fat, as shown in the diagram opposite. As a result, breakdown products called ketones are made which, although not harmful in small quantities, are poisonous acids in large amounts. One of the ketones, acetone (which smells like nail varnish remover), can be detected on the breath of some people with uncontrolled diabetes.

Ketones are danger signals, indicating virtual absence of insulin. After several hours of severe lack of insulin, large amounts of ketones give rise to the very serious condition of diabetic ketoacidosis. This is particularly likely to occur if insulin is reduced or stopped, or if you are vomiting or ill; it does not occur if you are eating and drinking normally.

Symptoms of this condition include:

- Confusion
- Weakness
- Increased passage of urine
- Excessive thirst
- Nausea
- Vomiting
- Abdominal upsets
- Shortness of breath.

If ketoacidosis remains untreated – and hospital treatment is always essential when this state has been reached – diabetic coma will follow. This carries significant risk. However, if you follow your treatment regime carefully, this condition should not occur. If it does, hospital treatment is nearly always successful.

EFFECT OF SEVERE INSULIN DEFICIENCY

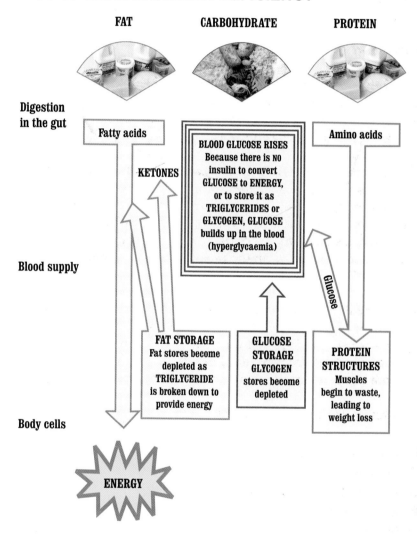

Breakdown of body energy stores. Because of a shortage of insulin and a consequent shortage of energy, alternative energy sources are provided by the breakdown of body energy stores (compare with the diagram on page 11)

Remember, once you have started insulin treatment, it should NEVER be stopped. It is absolutely ESSENTIAL that you PREVENT the risk of ketosis by taking enough insulin. Also, because illness can cause ketoacidosis, you should read carefully the section on how to deal with your diabetes when you are unwell (see page 110).

Other effects of high blood glucose

These include:

- ■ Infections: In the presence of high blood glucose, some other mechanisms in the body may not function as well as they should. During such periods you may be more prone to infections, such as abscesses, whitlows or urinary infections.
- ■ Blurring of vision: The high level of glucose in the body causes the lens of the eye to change slightly in shape. Consequently, short-sightedness is sometimes experienced when diabetes develops. The reverse sometimes occurs, making reading difficult. These changes may only be noticed in the early stages of treatment, and normally resolve completely in two or three weeks. It is wise, therefore, not to have your eyes tested for new glasses for at least one month after proper stabilisation of the diabetes.

■ Why treatment and good control of glucose need to be maintained

As indicated above, insulin treatment must be kept going to prevent ketoacidosis.

However, over a long period of time, a high blood glucose – even if it is not causing symptoms – will damage the small blood vessels in a number of tissues, the most commonly affected being:

- ■ The eyes – perhaps causing loss of vision
- ■ The nerves – causing numbness or painful tingling
- ■ The kidneys
- ■ The feet – especially in the elderly.

These are the so-called 'long-term' or 'late' complications of diabetes. They are discussed in more detail in Chapter 8.

It must be stressed that these complications will develop if a high blood glucose is sustained over a period of several years. Keeping your blood glucose close to normal largely eliminates the risk of these complications.

The only way to eliminate symptoms, prevent ketosis, and minimise late complications, is to commence treatment as soon as possible and to maintain it without interruption, keeping your blood glucose as close to normal as possible. You need to learn how to achieve this.

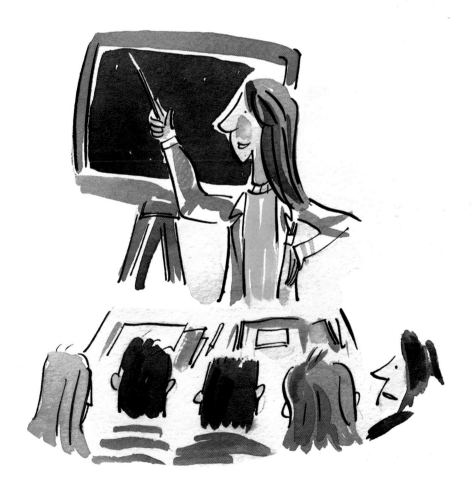

3 Controlling Your Diabetes

The main aims of treatment are to:

1. Eliminate symptoms.
2. Prevent late complications.
3. Allow life to be as full and normal as possible.

This chapter describes the main features of your treatment. These include:

- How insulin is administered.
- The types of insulin that you might use, and how they work.
- An outline of the different ways of using insulin.
- The adjustments you may need to make, to what and when you eat.
- Other factors likely to alter your blood glucose.

A more detailed description of fine tuning of your diabetes control is given in Chapter 5. Chapter 4 tells you how to find out how effective your control is. These general principles apply to all those receiving insulin treatment. Other chapters discuss diabetes in children (Chapter 10), pregnancy (Chapter 9) and older people who require insulin treatment (Chapter 11). However, because it deals with the basic principles, this chapter should be read before turning to the more specific chapters.

■ Eliminating symptoms

The first aim of treatment is to eliminate your symptoms. Once treatment has started, any feelings of thirst, excessive passage of urine, tiredness, weight loss, etc should disappear. As long as treatment is continued these symptoms should not recur.

■ Preventing late complications

If your blood glucose is returned to normal and kept there most of the time, the risk of complications will be very slight. Your treatment will need to be individually tailored to suit you. Unfortunately, there is no cure yet for diabetes, so the treatment must be continued. Needless to say, life is never constant, and your treatment will need to be adjusted to cope with, for example, job changes, pregnancy, retirement, etc.

However, you will soon recognise the factors that contribute to changes in your day-to-day blood glucose levels, such as your eating, working and exercise patterns. You should then be able to adjust your treatment accordingly, and maintain good control. In this way, what at first seems like a major upset will be under your control and adapted to suit your lifestyle.

In summary, the general principles of your treatment are four-fold:

1. You must take insulin injections to replace the insulin which you are failing to produce naturally – your insulin must never be stopped.
2. You must restore the balance between 'sugar in' and 'sugar out'. This will require you to make adjustments to the type and amount of food you eat, and when you eat it.
3. You should take some exercise if you are physically able to do so.
4. You must check that your treatment is effective.

■ Insulin

Injections of insulin

Unfortunately, there is no other way of giving insulin except by injection. Insulin cannot be given by mouth because it is a protein-like substance, which is destroyed in the stomach. Alternative methods are being investigated, eg inhaled insulin, but at present these are not yet sufficiently reliable to be recommended. Even if a pump is used the insulin is still delivered by a fine needle inserted under the skin. This has to be replaced regularly.

Initially, nearly everyone is apprehensive about having to inject themselves or their children with insulin. However, most people find the procedure to be simpler and much less painful than they first imagined.

Details of all you need to know about injections are given later in the chapter.

Insulin and restoring the balance

During the first few days of insulin injections, the aim will be to establish a balance between the insulin and blood glucose. The exact dose you need will be determined by the results of the tests you do. The point to remember is that you are trying to achieve small rises and falls in the glucose level in your blood, similar to those occurring normally. Your aim is to avoid wide swings in the blood glucose level.

Several factors may influence this balance:

- The type of insulin you inject
- The times of day at which you inject your insulin
- The site of injection
- The times at which you eat your meals
- The amount and type of food you eat
- The frequency, timing and quantity of exercise you take
- Stress and emotion
- Changes in bodyweight.

Overall targets of insulin control

The overall purpose of your treatment is to choose the timing and frequency of injection that keep your blood glucose at acceptable levels. You will be trying to avoid, therefore, high and low blood glucose levels. This does not mean that you will come to harm with occasional high levels. The overall purpose is to produce an average blood glucose which is acceptable. Clinics can now do tests to measure this average (see page 75). These tests, together with tests you can perform yourself, will help you achieve these aims.

Types of insulin

There are many types of insulin, each with different characteristics and varying length of action. Most insulin is now so-called 'human' insulin. This is not extracted from human pancreas, but is made in the laboratory. It is identical to that which occurs in the human body. Some 'pork' and 'beef' insulins are still available and they are extracted from the pancreas of pigs and cattle respectively. All insulins are highly purified, sterile, and free of any contamination.

VERY QUICK-ACTING ANALOGUE

NovoRapid (aspart)
Humalog (lispro)

CLEAR

QUICK-ACTING INSULINS/NEUTRAL INSULIN

Human Actrapid	Hypurin Bovine Neutral
Humaject S	Hypurin Porcine Neutral
Human Velosulin	Insuman Rapid
Humulin S	Pork Actrapid

CLEAR

MEDIUM- AND LONG-ACTING INSULINS

Human Insulated ge	Hypurin Porcine Isophane
Humulin I	Insuman Basal
Humulin Lente	Human Monotard
Humulin ZN	Pork Insulatard
Hypurin Bovine Isophane	Human Ultratard
Hypurin Bovine Lente	
Hypurin Bovine PZI	

CLOUDY

MIXED INSULINS

Humaject M3	Hypurin Porcine 30/70 mix
Human Mixtard 30,50	Insuman Comb 15
Human Mixtard 10, 20, 30, 40, 50	Insuman Comb 25
Humulin M3	Insuman Comb 50
Humulin M2	Pork Mixtard 30
Humulin M5	Humalog Mix 50
Humalog Mix 25, pen	

CLOUDY

Types of clear and cloudy insulin

The various insulins have minor differences in chemical structure but they all basically work in the same way.

When the pancreas is working normally, it produces short spurts or peaks of insulin in the blood after each meal or snack. However, when insulin is injected, its effect may last for only a few hours. Therefore an injection given before breakfast may no longer be active after lunch. A variety of insulins have been manufactured with different lengths of action. Some insulins are effective shortly after being injected, while others have a delayed action. Thus, by choosing the right type of insulin or mixture of insulins for you, normal, balanced spurts or peaks of insulin can be achieved.

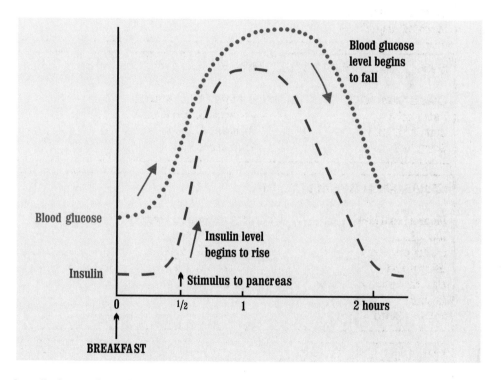

Insulin is produced after each meal or snack

So which insulin is best for you? This is a difficult question to answer. Some insulins work better and last for longer or shorter periods in different people. To start with you will be advised to take insulin which works reasonably well for most people. This treatment usually soon gets rid of all your symptoms. Then there will be a period of fine tuning, when, with results of your tests and discussions with your doctor, it may be decided that a change in type, timing or dose of insulin is better for you.

This 'trial and error' is essential to match your individual needs. No harm will come to you during short periods of less than perfect control. For complications to develop many years of poor control are needed.

Quick- and slow-acting insulins

The various types of insulin can be divided into four kinds:

1. Very quick-acting insulin (this is clear to the eye).
2. Quick-acting insulin (this is always clear to the eye).
3. Slow-acting insulin (this is always cloudy).
4. Mixtures of quick- and slow-acting insulins (these are also cloudy).

To check which insulins are which, look at the list on page 28.

Very quick-acting insulins

These insulins start working within a few minutes of injection. The maximum action occurs 30 to 60 minutes later. The effects usually wear off after 3 hours or so.

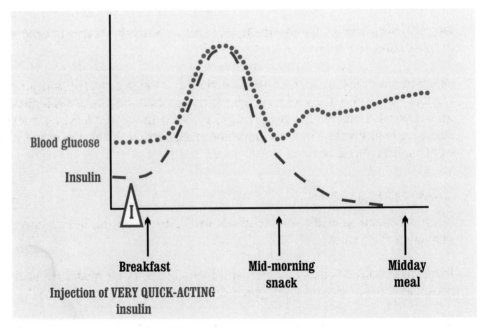

Very quick-acting insulin usually reaches its maximum 1 hour after a meal but wears off after 3 to 4 hours

Quick-acting insulins

These usually start working approximately 30 minutes after injected. They peak at 1 to 2 hours later. The effects usually last from 4 to 6 hours but may last for 8 to 10 hours.

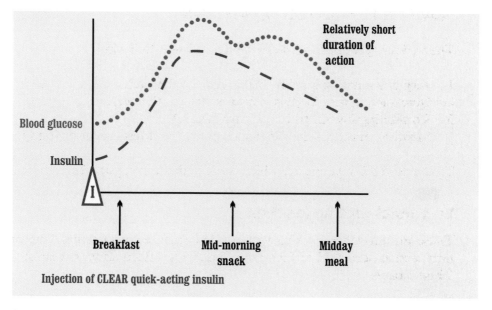

Relatively short duration of action

Blood glucose

Insulin

I

Breakfast   Mid-morning snack   Midday meal

Injection of CLEAR quick-acting insulin

Quick-acting insulin. Quick-acting insulin has a relatively short duration of action, lasting for 3 to 6 hours

You will remember that when the pancreas is working normally and producing its own insulin, the insulin level is highest when the glucose is highest, ie after a meal. Thus, with quick-acting insulin in the example given, most of the dose is available when it is most needed, namely, when the glucose has built up after breakfast.

Slow-acting insulins

Most slow-acting insulins usually last for 12 to 14 hours. Some, however, may last for 24 hours.

If injected before breakfast, they build slowly up. Their peaks are likely to coincide with the rise in blood glucose which follows the midday meal.

Some insulin does enter the blood stream earlier than this and remains there until late afternoon, thereby providing a small amount of insulin between the meals. Remember, a healthy pancreas supplies peak levels of insulin immediately after meals and a background level between meals. Slow-acting insulin is good for providing the trickle or background level, in order to hold the blood glucose steady between meals and overnight.

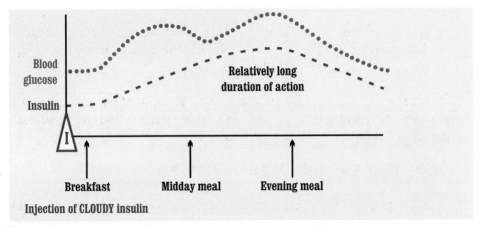

Blood glucose
Insulin
Relatively long duration of action
Breakfast   Midday meal   Evening meal
Injection of CLOUDY insulin

Slow-acting insulin. Slow-acting insulin is cloudy and has a relatively long duration of action

Mixtures of quick- and slow-acting insulin

A variety of different mixtures of quick- and slow-acting insulin are produced. These should enable you to combine the quick effect of the clear insulin and the longer effect of the slower-acting cloudy insulin to give you adequate insulin levels throughout the day. This can be necessary if it is found that your quick-acting insulin does not last long enough. Alternatively, if you are on just a slow-acting insulin, it may not work soon enough.

If you look at the graphs of how long the different insulins last and the effects on the blood glucose you will realise that a single injection of just one type of insulin is unlikely to control your blood sugar throughout the day.

The dose of insulin

In addition to the actual type of insulin, ie quick or slow, there is another factor to be considered – the dose.

The points to remember are that:

■ If the blood glucose is consistently high, larger doses of insulin are required.

- If the blood glucose is too low, smaller doses are required.
- The bigger the dose, the higher the level of insulin in the blood and the longer it takes to disappear, ie it lasts longer.

1. A large dose of QUICK-ACTING insulin lasts longer than a small dose.
2. A large dose of QUICK-ACTING insulin may last nearly as long as a small dose of SLOW-ACTING insulin.

This may seem very confusing, but once you establish your own pattern, with the help and advice of your doctor or specialist nurse – you will find that you can cope with almost any situation.

Choosing the right type of insulin

Quick-acting and slow-acting insulins can be used in many different ways to control diabetes. Slow-acting insulin provides a reasonable amount of background insulin but not much of a peak (see graph on page 32). This may occasionally work on its own in the early stages of treatment. This is because you may still be producing some insulin of your own.

However, for most people, some quick-acting insulin is required before breakfast and the main evening meal. This usually copes with the peaks of glucose that occur after these meals. The breakfast dose may, if it lasts long enough, also cover the peak of blood glucose after lunch. The second injection is then required before tea or supper to last through the night.

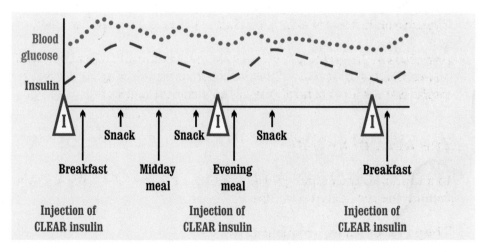

Twice-daily injections of quick-acting insulin

If you should only take one dose of slow-acting insulin in the morning a shortage of insulin during the night usually results. If the insulin dose is increased in the morning in order to produce higher levels during the evening and night, there may be too much present during the day. This situation is illustrated in the upper of the two diagrams below. This problem may be overcome by simply dividing this single dose of slow-acting insulin into two equal-sized injections. Smaller doses are shorter-acting.

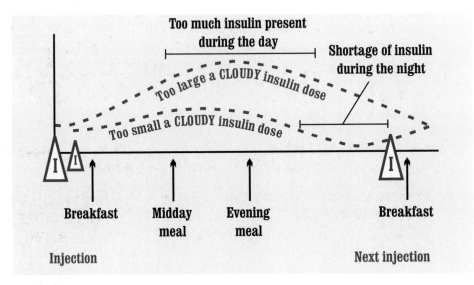

What happens if only a single, daily dose of slow-acting insulin is used

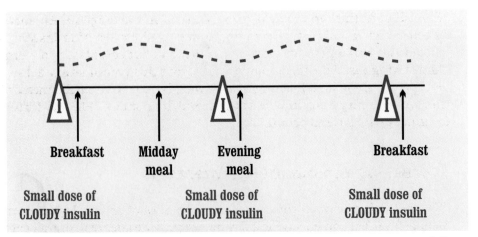

Smaller doses of slow-acting insulin are shorter-acting than a single, daily dose. By giving two injections it may be possible to ensure the necessary levels of insulin later in the day

One way to get these peaks and still keep a steady background trickle, is to take two injections, each combining quick- and slow-acting insulin. This adds up to the equivalent of four doses of insulin, each providing approximately a quarter of the daily requirement – smaller doses are shorter-acting.

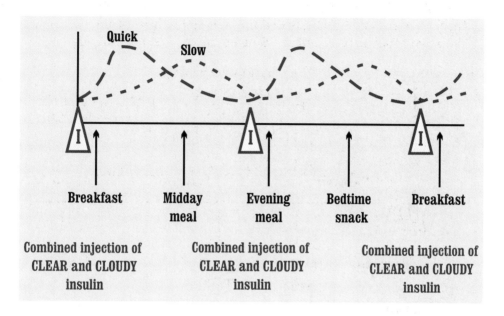

A combination of quick-acting and slow-acting insulins ensures peak as well as background levels of insulin

The effect of this type of dosage can be seen in the diagram. An injection taken before breakfast, combining quick- and slow-acting insulin, will provide an initial peak of quick-acting insulin after breakfast and a peak of slow-acting insulin after lunch. By repeating this combination before the evening meal, the quick-acting insulin will give a peak after the meal, while the slow-acting insulin will cover a bedtime snack. This will provide overnight background action.

Increasing the number of injections

The methods described above work for quite a lot of people. However, many people find that two injections a day do not provide adequate overall control. They do not allow sufficient variation for differences in timing and size of meals or snacks. The ideal way to cope with this is to increase the number of injections. By taking QUICK-ACTING before each meal (maybe three times a day) and SLOW-ACTING at night you can reproduce an insulin pattern which is very similar to that in someone without diabetes, ie peaks of insulin to cope with each meal and a steady trickle of background insulin in between (especially overnight).

Problems with mixtures of quick- and slow-acting insulins at night

As stated previously, ordinary quick-acting insulins may last for 6 hours or even longer. Let's examine what can happen if you take quick-acting insulin mixed with slow-acting insulin before your evening meal, say at 7 pm. The quick-acting insulin may be still present in considerable quantities at 1–3 am. At this time the slow-acting insulin is building up. This may lead to too high a level and the blood sugar will go too low (see hypoglycaemia).

The solution here is to use very quick-acting insulin before the evening meal. This will have disappeared from the blood in 3 to 4 hours (by bedtime) and this problem should not occur.

Summary

You will now realise that insulin can be used in many different ways. These include:

- Slow-acting insulin once daily
- Quick-acting insulin twice daily
- Slow-acting insulin twice daily
- Quick- or very quick and slow-acting insulin twice daily
- Slow-acting insulin once daily, quick-acting insulin twice daily
- Quick- or very quick-acting insulin several times a day before meals with slow-acting insulin overnight.

The choice of type will depend entirely on your individual needs. People often start with quick-acting insulin twice a day. This helps to get rid of your symptoms quickly and enables you to find out how this insulin works for you. Alternatives will then be chosen, once it is clear how you are getting on.

Timing of insulin injections

You have already seen how often injections should be given in order to cope with:

- The rise in blood glucose that occurs after each meal.
- The need for some insulin when you are not eating, between meals and overnight.

The quick-acting insulin is largely designed to cope with the peaks after meals and the slow-acting insulin to provide the trickle of background insulin between meals.

If you are taking twice-daily quick- or slow-acting insulin injections you should give the injections before your breakfast and before your evening meal.

If you are having more than two injections a day, the quick-acting insulin should be given 20–30 minutes before each meal and the slow-acting insulin usually at night (some people find that they need two injections of slow-acting, one at night and one in the morning).

Very quick-acting insulins must be given immediately before eating. Again, although this sounds complicated, you will soon know which suits you best.

Method of injection

Insulin injections can be given in three different ways:

- Using a standard syringe with an attached very fine needle
- Using a pen device
- By infusion pump.

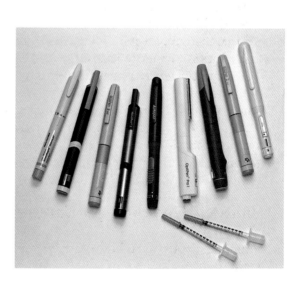

Standard syringe and examples of pen devices

Standard syringe

The syringe is small with a very fine needle. There are syringes of different sizes to cater for those using small, medium or large doses. There are also syringes with different length needles, eg very short for children, longer for adults. You fill the syringe from a bottle of insulin. You do, therefore, have to measure the dose yourself. You can use premixed or make up your own mixtures of quick- and slow-acting insulin. You will normally be taught this standard procedure in the first instance. It is usually the most convenient for those on one or two injections.

Pen devices

A number of so-called pen devices are available for injecting insulin. These contain a cartridge of insulin. The needles are provided separately and you have to attach one of these to the device. They all have a system where you set a dial to give the exact dose that you require. You then insert the needle in the normal way, as with the standard syringe, and press the plunger. This automatically delivers the right dose of insulin. These devices have the advantage that they are very portable. They contain enough insulin for several doses. You can carry them around in a pocket or handbag without any difficulty. Pre-filled pens are useful for people who have sight or dexterity problems. They are ideal, therefore, for people using multiple injections, especially when they are giving an injection before each meal (more details of multiple injection techniques are provided in Chapter 6).

Pen or standard syringe?

This is normally a matter of personal choice. However, the cartridges used in pens are pre-filled with one type of insulin. If you are using a mixture of quick-acting and slow-acting insulin and, as is often the case, need to vary the amounts of quick and slow to cope with different daily activities, you therefore have to use a syringe.

Secondly, pens are bigger and slightly heavier. Some people, especially those with arthritis of the hands, sometimes find difficulty in pressing the plunger. Children may have difficulty as the pens may be rather cumbersome. On the other hand, pens may be much easier, particularly if you are travelling or need to give insulin from home. If you are using a mixture of quick and slow, there are ready-mixed insulins that can be used with pens, and these may suit you.

If in doubt, ask your specialist nurse or doctor.

Where is insulin given?

You can choose any of the injection sites shown in the diagram. You should use one site for the morning injection and a different site for the evening injection, for example, abdomen in the morning, legs in the evening. Vary the side as well, eg left on Monday, right on Tuesday, etc. Having chosen a general area, make sure that you vary the point of entry each day, otherwise you will develop a scar or fatty lump, which will prevent the insulin from being adequately absorbed.

The speed at which insulin works may vary according to the site of injection. A quicker response occurs after injecting in the abdomen than in the thighs.

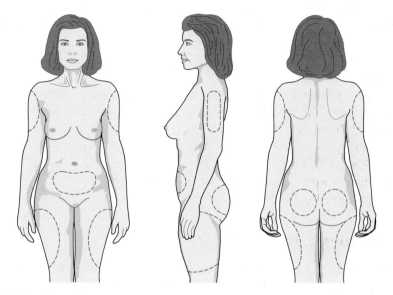

Where to inject insulin

Insulin infusion pumps

Infusion pumps have been developed in an attempt to avoid repeated injections of insulin. These are battery-driven and are worn on a belt or holster. The insulin is delivered via a fine tube connected to a needle. This needle is inserted under the skin of the abdomen. It may be left in the same place for several days. The pumps are designed to deliver a trickle of insulin continuously to provide the background insulin, but the user can trigger the delivery of an additional dose of insulin before each meal.

The pump would appear to provide insulin in a very similar way to the normal pancreas. However, they do have certain disadvantages. Many people find it irritating to always have the pump attached to them. Also the needle does have to be moved from time to time, so you do not avoid injections altogether. They are expensive and their maintenance may be difficult.

Of even greater importance, however, they may, like all mechanical devices, malfunction. Because they trickle insulin in very slowly, if the pump fails, the insulin levels in the blood may fall off very quickly. If the person does not realise that the pump has failed, ketosis may develop very rapidly (see page 110).

You have to appreciate that pumps are just an alternative way of giving insulin. You still have to work out how much insulin you need for each meal or snack. You also have to calculate how much insulin you need to trickle in between meals. To become confident about this does require a fairly intensive period of training.

You cannot just assume that the pump is going to control your diabetes on its own. You have to drive it. This does, of course, mean making the same sorts of decisions based on regular testing (see Chapter 4) as you do with ordinary injection treatment. If not, your diabetes control may get worse rather than better.

More information about pump therapy is provided in Chapter 6.

Worries about injections

Fear of giving injections

After giving your first injection, much of the fear will disappear. Like most people with diabetes, you will no doubt have been surprised that the injection was almost painless.

Spilling insulin

If insulin squirts out from around the needle when you press in the plunger, do not worry. It is important that you should not start all over again, unless you are sure that all the insulin has been wasted in this way. Rather than worry about whether you have taken in sufficient insulin, it is better and safer to pay particular attention to your test results. One faulty injection will not have serious consequences.

Swelling and pain at the injection site

It is quite common for a little redness to develop at the site of the injection. This may persist for a day or two when you first start injections, but it usually disappears after a week or so. Occasionally you may develop little blisters when you inject, usually because you are not injecting deeply enough. If after injecting more deeply you still develop blisters, tell your doctor.

Infection at the injection site

Infection of this nature is very rare. With reasonable cleanliness – you don't need a gown and gloves – this should never occur.

Some commonly asked questions about injections

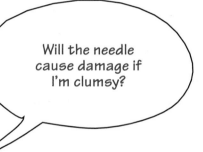

Will the needle cause damage if I'm clumsy?

No. If you inject where you are shown to inject, you can't do any damage.

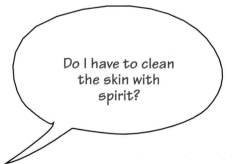

Do I have to clean the skin with spirit?

No, this merely hardens the skin. As long as the skin is clean, no swabbing with spirit is necessary.

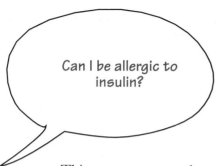

Can I be allergic to insulin?

This occurs very rarely and will be obvious to your doctor at the outset. Even if you are allergic, the problem can be readily overcome by changing to another type of insulin.

Care of equipment

Disposal of syringes, pen needles and lancets

What to do with old syringes, needles and lancets can be a problem for people with Type 1 diabetes, since you cannot just throw them away in the dustbin. The following are simple guidelines for the safe disposal of your sharps.

1. Use the BD Safe-clip, which is available on prescription, to shear off the syringe/pen needle. This gadget will hold approximately 200 needles and when full can safely be thrown in the dustbin.

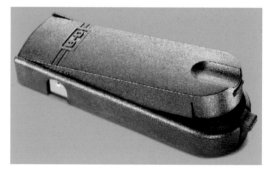

Getting rid of old syringes

2. Place the shaft of the syringe into a rigid container with a lid, eg a bleach bottle. When the container is full, tape the top to make sure it is secure and put it into the dustbin. These guidelines are to be followed with agreement from your local authority refuse department.

You may also be able to obtain a 'sharps bin' from your doctor.

Reusing disposable needles

These are intended to be used only once, as reusing needles can lead to blunting of the needle, the needle becoming blocked if you use mixed insulin, and the needle becoming brittle and so breaking more easily; and the needle's lubricant lasts for just one injection.

Reusing disposable syringes

Like disposable needles, these are normally intended to be used once only. It is quite safe to use these syringes more than once, however, as long as the markings do not become so worn that it is difficult to measure the dose accurately. If you decide to use a disposable syringe more than once, then after each injection cover the needle with its sterile cap, and keep it in a refrigerator.

Occasionally needles become blocked, especially very fine ones. To check for a blockage, work the plunger in and out and if resistance is felt or if it is very difficult to draw up the insulin, discard the needle and use another.

After use always put the cap back on the needle. Change the needle when it gets blunt. Do not try to wash disposable syringes. They can be used more than once, but change them if the markings are worn.

Pens

These are very robust and can be carried in a pocket or handbag. Change the needle when it gets blunt.

■ Timing of meals

Meals provide the blood glucose peaks already mentioned. Therefore, the timing of insulin injections in relation to your meals is important.

THE TIMING OF MEALS IN RELATION TO INSULIN INJECTIONS

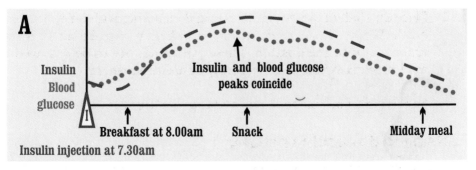

Meal taken at least half an hour after insulin injection

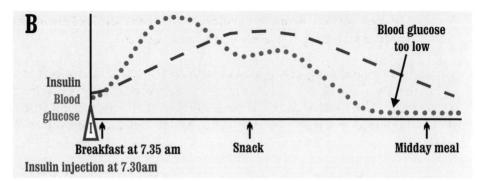

Meal taken only a few minutes after quick-acting insulin injection

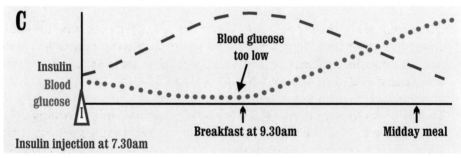

Meal delayed for two hours after insulin injection

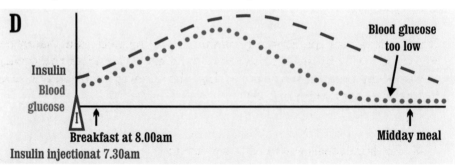

Mid-morning snack omitted

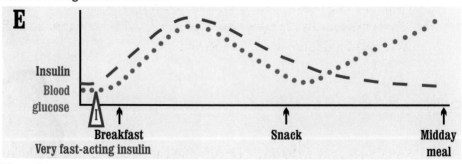

The effect of a quick-acting insulin

Blood glucose control will only be achieved if the peak levels of insulin in the blood coincide with the peak levels of glucose (panel A).

If you inject standard quick-acting insulin only a few minutes before your meal, the insulin peak will occur some time after your glucose peak, because of the time taken for the insulin to be absorbed. As a consequence you may have a high mid-morning glucose level and a low late morning glucose level (panel B).

If after having injected your insulin you delay eating your meal by, say, two hours, the insulin peak will occur well before the glucose peak (panel C).

Quite frequently, the glucose provided by your main meals may not last long enough. Two or three hours after a meal, your glucose level may be falling but your insulin level may still be quite high. If no steps are taken to counter this, your blood glucose may fall too low (panel D).

To avoid this, top up blood glucose levels by eating a mid-morning or mid-afternoon snack, and perhaps taking a snack before you go to bed at night. This is often recommended in the initial stages of treatment, though you may find, as you get more experienced, that you can cut these down or do without them.

If you take a very quick-acting insulin, this is injected immediately before the meal. Your blood glucose may be reasonable after the meal; but because the insulin is shorter acting, the blood glucose may rise again before the next meal (panel E).

- For large meals you need more insulin.
- For small meals less insulin is required.
- You may need more insulin for some types of food.
- If you miss meals after your injection you will have too much insulin and the blood glucose will go too low.

■ Diet

The remainder of the chapter decribes the eating habits and food choices that are best for people with diabetes.

What will the diet be like?

Food recommended for people with diabetes is not a special diet as such. It may not be very different from your present diet. It is, in fact, a healthy way of eating that can be recommended for everyone.

However, it is particularly important for those taking insulin for the following reasons:

- ▉ If the diet contains too much high sugar food you will have difficulty controlling your blood glucose levels.
- ▉ By eating regular meals and snacks containing plenty of starchy foods like bread, pasta, rice, potatoes, chapattis, cassava and cereals you will avoid low blood glucose levels (hypoglycaemia).
- ▉ Eating a well balanced, healthy diet will help reduce the risks of other problems with your health in later life.
- ▉ It is always sensible to try to maintain a normal weight, but particularly if you have diabetes.

Finally, once you have taken your insulin you do have to have something to eat and may need a snack 2–3 hours later. Greater attention than usual is therefore necessary to the timing of meals and snacks.

Food plays a very important part in our lives and therefore making changes to our diet can affect more than just meal times. Our eating patterns and the types of food we eat are often a lifelong habit. Good habits established early will help you later in life.

Any changes which are recommended will help you with your diabetes control. They should also allow flexibility to fit in with your daily lifestyle and allow you to eat as varied and interesting meals as normal. You can achieve this more easily if you understand the basic principles. The next section describes the basic components of food and explains the various terms used to describe them. This is followed by advice on how you can make simple changes to help your diabetes control.

The basic components of food

Our food falls into three main groups – carbohydrate, protein and fat. They are all essential for a balanced diet. Most foods contain mixtures of one or more of these nutrients. For example, milk contains carbohydrate, protein and fat; eggs contain fat and protein, and pastry is mainly fat and carbohydrate. In general, vegetables and fruit contain little or no fat, while cheese, margarine and meat contain no carbohydrate.

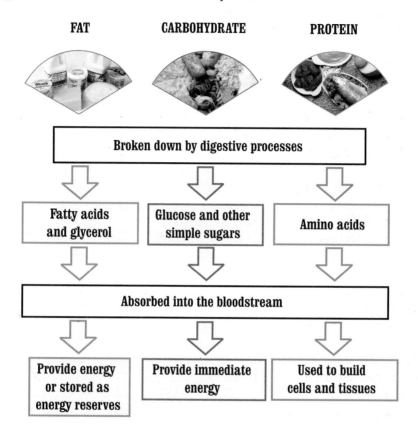

The three basic constituents of food

Carbohydrate

Carbohydrate is found in starchy and sugary foods.

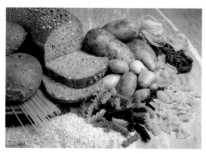

Some typical carbohydrate-
containing foods

All carbohydrates are broken down in the body to glucose (sugar) and so will cause the blood glucose level to rise. Choose starchy foods, eg bread, potatoes, breakfast cereals, rice, chapattis, cassava, yam and pasta as the basis of all meals and snacks even if you are watching your weight. Eating starchy foods regularly helps blood glucose control. This is the reason why meals should be based on these types of foods.

Glucose is essential for the body to function normally, and a reasonable supply is therefore necessary. However, very sugary foods, eg soft drinks and sweets, tend to be digested very quickly and cause a rapid and large increase in the blood glucose level. This increase may be short-lived and can produce swings from high to low. This may make it more difficult to control your diabetes.

Protein

Foods high in animal protein include meat, milk, eggs, fish and dairy products. Protein is essential in the diet, because it provides the building materials for the cells and tissues of the body. However, foods high in animal protein also tend to be high in fat. It is therefore wise not to eat large quantities of these. Vegetable sources of protein, eg cereals and pulses, are a low fat alternative to animal protein and are also a good source of soluble fibre (see page 50) This helps limit the rise in blood glucose after meals. Try to replace some of the animal protein in your diet with these foods.

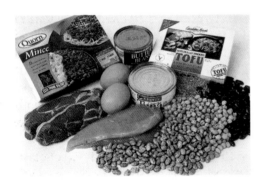

These foods are all sources of protein

Fat

Only small quantities of fat are necessary for good health. Obvious sources of fat are butter, margarine, oil, lard and dripping. Fatty meats and full-fat dairy products contain fat too. You should also watch out for the fat found in cakes, biscuits, snacks and pastries.

There are three types of fat:

- Saturated fats
- Polyunsaturated fats
- Monounsaturated fats.

They all contain the same amount of calories, but saturated fats particularly can raise blood cholesterol levels. Saturated fats are usually found in animal products, eg fatty meat, suet, lard, butter, cheese, milk and other full-fat dairy products.

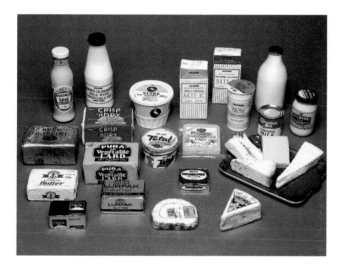

Foods high in fat

Unsaturated fats should be used in preference to foods high in saturated fats. When choosing a cooking oil, select those which state on the label that they are high in monounsaturated or polyunsaturated fats. Monounsaturated fats are found in olive and rapeseed oil. They have been shown to improve blood cholesterol levels. Oily fish, eg herring, tuna and mackerel, are particularly recommended. These contain a type of polyunsaturated fat which also helps keep cholesterol levels down. Try to eat this type of fish at least once a week.

It is not the amount of cholesterol in the food which affects blood cholesterol. Everybody has cholesterol in their blood. It forms an important part of cells and tissues. Unfortunately too much cholesterol can lead to a build up of fatty deposits in the arteries. Most cholesterol in the body is made from other food – especially saturated fat. Some foods are naturally high in cholesterol. Cutting down on these has a limited effect. The most benefit is achieved by eating less saturated fat. Cholesterol also rises as you become overweight. Weight control will therefore help to keep levels down.

It is important to remember that all types of fat are high in calories, and only small quantities should be used. Whenever possible, try to choose monounsaturated or polyunsaturated fats in preference to saturated ones.

Fibre

Dietary fibre is a substance of plant origin which is not broken down in the human digestive system. It is good for helping to lower your blood glucose levels as well as helping to prevent constipation. High-fibre foods also tend to be bulky, so they fill you up more quickly – this is especially important if you are trying to lose weight.

There are two types of fibre: insoluble and soluble. Insoluble fibre helps the prevention of constipation. Foods containing soluble fibre tend to have less effect on the rise in blood sugar and are therefore good for your blood glucose levels. Fruits and vegetables, and the outside coats of grains and cereals, all contain fibre.

Insoluble fibre is found in wheat bran, wholemeal flour, wholemeal bread, brown pasta and brown rice.

Foods that are high in soluble fibre are, for example, fruit and vegetables, peas, beans, oats and lentils. They slow down the rise in blood glucose levels after a meal.

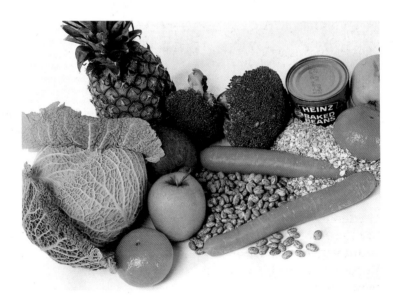

Foods high in soluble fibre

Remember that you do not have to eat wholemeal foods all the time, but try to include a variety of high-fibre choices across the day.

Here are some ways to increase your fibre intake:

- Add extra vegetables and pulses to soups and casseroles.
- Instead of white flour, use wholemeal flour or a mixture of half white and half wholemeal.
- Leave the skin on potatoes.
- Eat the skin of jacket and boiled potatoes.
- Add dried fruits to puddings, cakes and biscuits.
- Snack on fruit.
- Eat fruit-based puddings.
- Add pulses and pasta to salads.
- Add peas and/or sweetcorn to rice during cooking.
- Try a variety of breads, including wholemeal or granary.

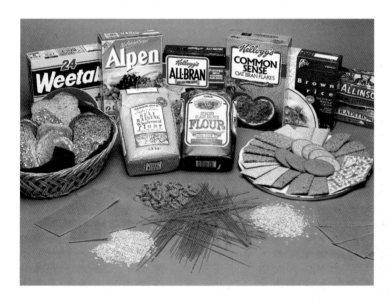

Foods high in insoluble fibre

Vitamins and minerals

There are many vitamins and minerals and they are all vital for good health. If you are eating the right balance of carbohydrate, protein and fat, and plenty of fruit and vegetables, then adequate amounts of vitamins and minerals should automatically be included in the diet. Supplements should not therefore be necessary.

■ Healthy eating – putting it into practice

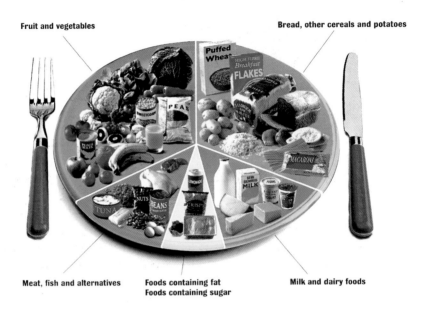

Fruit and vegetables   Bread, other cereals and potatoes

Meat, fish and alternatives   Foods containing fat   Milk and dairy foods
                                   Foods containing sugar

The balance of good health

In order to make the right choices it is easiest to think of meals as a whole. To do this, consider a plate of food. This is likely to consist of foods falling into five main groups:

- Starchy carbohydrate, eg bread, potatoes, rice, pasta, cereals, chapattis, cassava, yam.
- Fruit and vegetables.
- Meat, poultry, fish, eggs or meat alternative (for example, beans and pulses).
- Dairy foods – milk, cheese, yogurts.
- High fat and high sugar foods, eg jam, honey, butter, margarine, oils.

As explained in the previous section, you need to get a balance so that your plate contains a relatively high proportion of starchy carbohydrate and fruit and vegetables, with small amounts of meat and fish (or alternatives) and milk and dairy foods. High fat and high sugar foods should be limited to small amounts.

Starchy carbohydrate

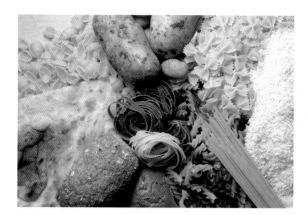

Examples of starchy carbohydrates

- Starchy carbohydrate foods are broken down to glucose, for energy.
- Your diet must therefore contain enough carbohydrate to ensure a reasonable level of blood glucose in order to produce the fuel your body needs.
- Each of your meals should be based mainly on starchy foods, as the plate model shows. If you feel hungry between meals, choose snacks that contain starchy carbohydrate such as bread or rolls and cereals.
- You should not cut out foods containing carbohydrate. This would merely encourage your body to produce more glucose from its reserves, which would cause you to lose weight and become unwell. Starvation is no treatment for diabetes.
- Starchy foods which are high in fibre, especially soluble fibre, eg pasta, help slow down the rise in blood glucose further and are therefore good choices to include in your diet.

How much carbohydrate?

Diabetes is about balance. You need to balance your insulin with the carbohydrate foods in your diet (which raise your blood glucose) and daily activity (which lowers your blood glucose).

You will therefore need a reasonable helping of starchy carbohydrate for each meal. The quantity should be spread fairly evenly over the main meals, with additional snacks containing starchy carbohydrate between meals if you need them.

In the past the amount of carbohydrate recommended was counted using an exchange system. The idea was to spread the carbohydrate across the day and keep the carbohydrate content of each meal and snack about the same. Lists of carbohydrate foods were provided showing the amounts containing 10 g of carbohydrate, for example:

1 small, thin slice wholemeal bread = 10 g carbohydrate

1 Weetabix = 10 g carbohydrate

4 tablespoons baked beans = 10 g carbohydrate

This system assumed that all the foods on the list would affect the blood glucose in exactly the same way. However, this is not the case. Some carbohydrate foods are absorbed much more rapidly than others. Those that are absorbed quickly increase the blood glucose level faster. For example, 100 ml of fresh orange juice and one large orange both contain the same amount of carbohydrate, but their effect on your blood glucose will be different.

To help you judge which carbohydrates have the greater or lesser effect a grading system has been developed, called the glycaemic index (GI). The most rapidly absorbed carbohydrate is glucose, which is pure sugar. Those foods which have a similar effect to glucose are said to have a high glycaemic index. Pulses, eg lentils and butter beans, on the other hand, are absorbed very slowly, causing a gentle rise in blood glucose. They are therefore said to have a low glycaemic index. Examples are listed on the next page.

Combining foods of high glycaemic index with those with a low index will help reduce the rise in blood glucose after meals. For example, you can try combining mashed potatoes (high) with baked beans (low) or cornflakes (moderatly high) with fruit (low). This will enable you to have varied meals and continue to eat things that you enjoy and control your blood glucose levels more easily.

You cannot tell a low GI food just by looking at it – and GI is not just related to the fibre or sugar content of a food. The effect on blood glucose levels of a meal or snack is influenced by many things. The way in which a food is cooked and prepared, the other constituents of the meal and their fat and protein content, as well as different foods you have eaten that day can all have a bearing on its GI. It is not possible at the moment, therefore, to label all the foods we might eat according to their GI.

You do not need to exclude all foods with a high GI and eat only foods with a low GI. To apply the benefits of GI to your diet, however, try to include low GI foods with each meal, which lowers the overall glycaemic effect of a meal. Low GI foods like fruit and vegetables, beans and pulses, pasta and oats form part of a well balanced diet anyway.

The best way to apply information about glycaemic index is to combine fruit, vegetables and pulses with meals and snacks in order to help you to control blood glucose levels more easily. This also fits in with Healthy Eating guidelines. However, by checking your own blood glucose responses to different meals you will soon learn what suits you and your diabetes control best.

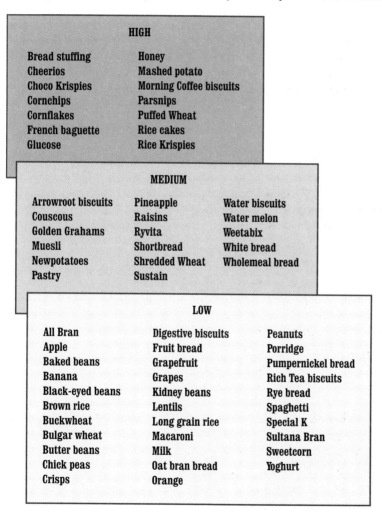

HIGH

Bread stuffing	Honey
Cheerios	Mashed potato
Choco Krispies	Morning Coffee biscuits
Cornchips	Parsnips
Cornflakes	Puffed Wheat
French baguette	Rice cakes
Glucose	Rice Krispies

MEDIUM

Arrowroot biscuits	Pineapple	Water biscuits
Couscous	Raisins	Water melon
Golden Grahams	Ryvita	Weetabix
Muesli	Shortbread	White bread
Newpotatoes	Shredded Wheat	Wholemeal bread
Pastry	Sustain	

LOW

All Bran	Digestive biscuits	Peanuts
Apple	Fruit bread	Porridge
Baked beans	Grapefruit	Pumpernickel bread
Banana	Grapes	Rich Tea biscuits
Black-eyed beans	Kidney beans	Rye bread
Brown rice	Lentils	Spaghetti
Buckwheat	Long grain rice	Special K
Bulgar wheat	Macaroni	Sultana Bran
Butter beans	Milk	Sweetcorn
Chick peas	Oat bran bread	Yoghurt
Crisps	Orange	

Examples of foods with high, medium and low glycaemic index

Fruit and vegetables

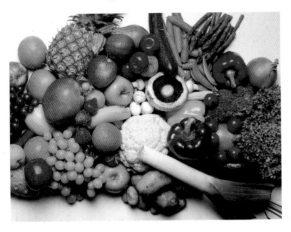

**Fruit and vegetables are
essential for a healthy diet**

Fruit and vegetables should also be included in your diet in generous portions. A good guide is to include at least five servings of fruit or vegetables each day. They contain vitamins and fibre which help to even out blood glucose levels.

Remember, frozen and canned fruit in natural juice and vegetables are good alternatives to fresh. Try to have fruit and vegetables at each meal. Fruit is an ideal between-meal snack.

Meat, fish, eggs and pulses

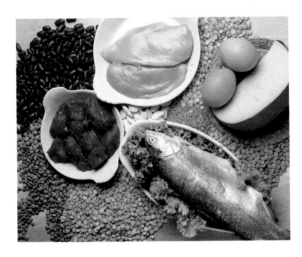

Foods rich in protein

These foods provide the body with protein.

- To keep down the saturated fat in your diet, choose lean red meat and remove the skin from poultry. Grill rather than fry meat products including burgers and sausages.
- Include more white fish, which is lower in fat than meat, in your diet. Oily fish such as tuna, salmon, sardines, mackerel and pilchards are high in fat, but it is the kind of fat that helps to protect you from heart disease. Aim to eat fish at least twice a week.
- Alternatives to meat such as peas, beans and lentils are a good source of protein but are low in fat. They also have a low glycaemic effect. Try replacing some of the meat in your diet with some of these.
- Soya products, such as tofu, and other vegetarian alternatives like Quorn are also low in fat and can be used to replace meat in cooking.

Milk and dairy foods

Full-fat milk and dairy foods contain a lot of saturated fat which can raise blood cholesterol. You can keep the fat down but still get the calcium you need by:

- Using semi-skimmed or skimmed milk
- Choosing low fat yoghurts
- Saving cream and cream products for special occasions
- Eating lower fat hard cheeses or cottage cheese in place of full fat varieties.

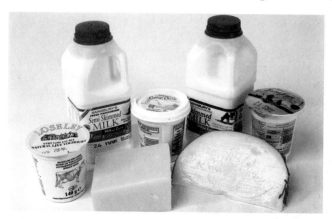

A daily intake of three servings will provide you with all the calcium that you need. A serving is one-third of a pint of milk, one pot of yoghurt or a piece of cheese the size of a small matchbox.

Keeping down the fat in your diet

It is perfectly acceptable to have some fat and sugar as part of a balanced diet. However, too much fatty food should be avoided. Here are some guidelines to follow:

- Cut down on fatty foods and use less fat and oil in cooking.
- Use monounsaturated oils, such as olive oil or rapeseed oil, rather than saturated fats such as butter and lard.
- Try not to have high fat snacks such as crisps, cakes and biscuits every day.
- Reduced fat and fat-free products can be tried.

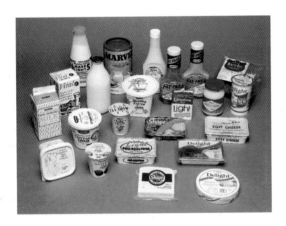

Reduced fat and fat-free products

More about sugar

High sugar foods should also be kept to a minimum. They cause a rapid rise in your blood glucose, and can be high in fat and calories, and are best limited if you are watching your weight. Drinks which contain a lot of sugar are best replaced with a sugar-free alternative. However, as long as your day-to-day eating is healthy and your diabetes is well controlled, foods which contain some sugar like cakes and biscuits are perfectly acceptable choices.

Sweet foods which normally put the blood glucose up quickly when eaten on their own, are less likely to do so if you have already eaten a meal. For example, you can try small amounts of sweet foods such as chocolate after a main course of vegetable stir fry. If you eat too much in your diet, you will not be eating a healthy balanced diet and are more likely to become overweight. Here are some guidelines to follow:

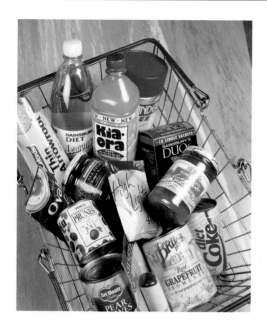

A wide range of low sugar and
sugar-free products is available

- Try low sugar and sugar-free foods such as sugar-free jelly and sugar-free instant puddings, which many supermarkets now sell.
- Diet or 'light' foods contain less sugar as well as less fat, for example tinned milk puddings and custard.
- If a food or drink is labelled as 'no added sugar', this does not mean that it is sugar-free. For example, unsweetened fruit juice has no sugar added to it but it contains a lot of sugar naturally.
- The sorts of foods that you should restrict are those which are obviously very sweet. There are, however, times when you will definitely need something sweet.

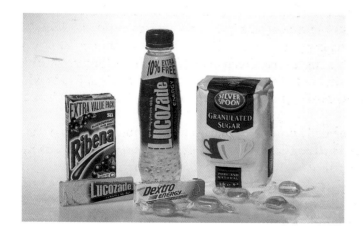

Foods high in sugar
should be restricted

When you must take something sweet

On occasions you will need to push your blood glucose up to avoid hypogly-caemia. Exercise burns up sugar more quickly. Before heavy exercise, sport or manual work you may find it necessary to take some extra carbohydrate, eg a cereal bar (see page 189).

■ If you feel your blood glucose is going low, ie you are developing hypoglycaemia, you must immediately take some rapidly absorbed glucose. Sugar in liquid form, eg Lucozade, is most rapidly absorbed (see page 115).

What are sweeteners?

There are two main types of sweetener: non-intense and intense sweeteners.

Non-intense sweeteners

These include fructose and polyols (like sorbitol, maltitol, mannitol, isomalt, xylitol). They are sometimes known as nutritive or bulk sweeteners.

Non-intense sweeteners are not recommended as sweeteners. This is because they offer no benefit over ordinary sugar to people with diabetes. They contain calories and carbohydrate and so can still cause blood glucose levels to rise. They also have a laxative effect. Foods that contain a significant amount of non-intense sweeteners have to be labelled with a warning 'Excessive consumption may produce laxative effects'. Non-intense sweeteners are commonly used in diabetic foods, tooth friendly sweets and some sugar-free confectionery.

Fructose (fruit sugar) is sometimes used in foods such as low fat yoghurts as an alternative to sugar. Diabetes UK does not feel that fructose in foods offers any special advantage over sugar to people with diabetes. Everyday foods that contain fructose can be eaten, but fructose is not recommended as a table top sweetener or for use in cooking.

Intense sweeteners

Intense sweeteners are also known as artificial sweeteners. There are four types that are most commonly used in food products in this country: aspartame (Nutrasweet™), saccharin, acesulfame potassium (acesulfame K) and cyclamates. The intense sweetener used in a food will always be in the ingredients listing – either the name or additive number.

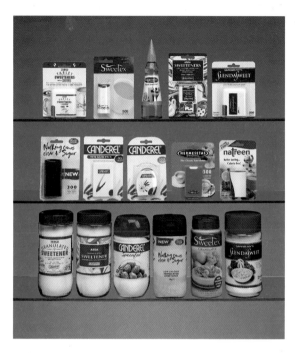

Intense sweeteners are both carbohydrate and calorie free. They will not affect blood glucose levels. Because they are very intense only small amounts need to be used. These sweeteners are used widely in manufactured foods and are also available as tablet, liquid and granulated sweeteners for use at home. They can be used in drinks, on cereals and in certain puddings if you require extra sweetness.

Intense sweeteners

Diabetic foods

There is no need to buy special 'diabetic' foods. They are expensive and will not help your diabetes.

Salt

Eating too much salt can lead some people to develop high blood pressure. It is sensible to cut down on the amount of salt in your diet.

- Reduce the amount of salt used in cooking and use less salt at the table.
- Tinned, packaged and processed foods tend to be higher in salt, so eat less of these.

Checking the label

What the terms mean

Energy: the amount of energy (calories) that a food provides. Look for the 'kcal' figure which means calories. To keep to a healthy weight, the energy we eat (found in calories) needs to balance with the amount of energy used in daily life.

Protein: protein is needed for growth and repair. Most adults eat more than enough protein so don't worry about this on the label.

Carbohydrate: the total carbohydrate in food, which includes sugars and starches. You should get most of the energy in your diet from starch. **Eat more**

'Of which sugars': the amount of the carbohydrate that is sugars – that's both natural and added sugars. **Eat less**

Fat: the total amount of fat in foods – polyunsaturated, monounsaturated and saturated fats. **Eat less**

'Of which saturates': the type of fat you need to particularly limit. **Eat less**

Fibre: fibre is important for a healthy bowel. **Eat more**

Sodium: indicates how much salt is in a food. **Eat less**

NUTRITION INFORMATION		
	per 100g	per 25g serving
ENERGY	1560 kj 367 kcal	390 kj 92 kcal
PROTEIN	7.3g	1.8g
CARBOHYDRATE of which sugars	82.7g 8.9g	20.7g 2.2g
FAT of which saturates	0.8g 0.3g	0.2g 0.1g
FIBRE	3.6g	0.9g
SODIUM	1.1g	0.3g

What the label tells you

Do the figures mean a lot or a little?

To judge whether a food contains a little or a lot of a nutrient, use the 'per 100g' figure for a snack food and the 'per serving' figure for a complete meal.

Energy: If you are overweight, you need to eat fewer calories and increase the amount of activity you do to use up more calories.

Sugar: 10g or more of sugar is a lot. 2g or less of sugar is a little.

Fat: 20g or more of fat is a lot. 3g or less of fat is a little.

Saturates: 5g or more is a lot. 1g or less is a little.

Fibre: 3g or more is a lot. 0.5g or less is a little.

Sodium: 0.5g or more is a lot. 0.1g or less is a little.

When you check food labels for sugar, you may be surprised to find that many foods contain sugar, from tinned vegetables and soups, sauces and pickles to bread and baked beans.

The amount of sugar present in such foods is often small and is unlikely to affect your blood glucose levels. Therefore you do not need to avoid such foods. As a general guide, look at the label – the lower down the list of ingredients sugar appears, the less there is present in the product.

The important thing to consider is how much of a particular food you eat, as well as how much fat or sugar it may contain.

When looking at labels it is easier to compare foods of similar type, eg look at labels of different types of biscuit. Choose those lower in sugar and fat and if possible higher in fibre.

Eating out

As your knowledge of healthy eating increases, you will gain more confidence when eating out, and you will be able to select those foods which you consider to be good combinations.

Eating with friends and relatives should pose no problems. If you let them know in advance which foods you prefer not to eat, any embarrassment will easily be avoided.

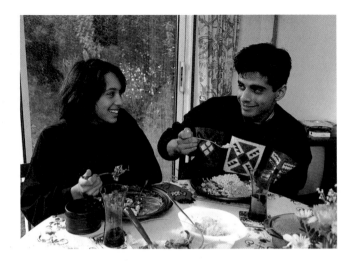

Whether eating out in pubs, Indian, Chinese, Italian or other restaurants, it is always possible to ensure that your meal contains plenty of carbohydrate. Such meals may be higher in fat than those you are used to, but you can choose the lower fat dishes.

Fast food – hamburgers, cheeseburgers, hot dogs and fish and chips – are usually very high in fat.

If you are at all concerned about the suitability of certain foods in a restaurant, do not be afraid to ask. Wherever possible:

- Select generous portions of vegetables and bread.
- Avoid too many fatty and high-sugar foods. (Choose sugar-free thirst-quenchers.)
- Choose baked, grilled and boiled foods as opposed to those that are fried or roasted.

However, if you only eat out occasionally, although it may lead to a temporary rise in blood glucose or a higher intake of fat, it will do no long-term harm.

Timing of meals

If you miss meals or snacks you run a significant risk of low blood glucose or hypoglycaemia. This risk can be reduced if you take frequent injections of short-acting insulin. The frequent injections allow you to delay the meal for an hour or so since you will also delay the insulin injection which you give just before it.

For many people who are still taking twice-daily insulin, delaying or missing a meal is likely to cause hypoglycaemia. Of course, there may be occasions when meals get unavoidably delayed. In this case, have a snack (a hunk of bread or a sandwich) to keep you going until you get your proper meal.

If you are due to take an insulin injection before the meal, do not take it until you know you are going to get something to eat half an hour or so after the injection.

Must I always take snacks?

This is again a question of trial and error and depends on the individual. If you are taking frequent injections just before meals snacks may not be necessary. If you are taking insulin which lasts longer, say twice a day, then you may find you do need snacks between meals to avoid going too low.

Weight concerns

If you have diabetes and are overweight, losing weight will benefit your general health and improve your diabetes control.

Some people can lose weight more quickly than others, but no one finds it easy. You have to look honestly at what you are eating and try to pinpoint areas where you could cut down. Are you eating lots of fatty foods, ie fatty meats, lots of butter, crisps, nuts, pastries and pies? Could you be making more use of low calorie or high fibre foods?

The type of diet you choose must be nutritionally balanced. Miracle diets and very low calorie diets can be tempting, but do not have long-term effects. They are very likely to cause difficulties with your blood glucose control. In particular the risk of hypoglycaemia will be high.

Losing weight takes time – you put weight on slowly and it takes a similar time to lose it again. Aim to lose a half to one kilogram (one to two pounds) each week. Because your weight fluctuates, you should not be tempted to weigh yourself every day. Instead, weigh yourself once a week, preferably on the same day and first thing in the morning.

Set yourself a realistic target weight. Aim for a moderate weight loss to start with and once you have achieved this, set a new target if necessary.

Adjusting your insulin when you are losing weight

When you are overweight you normally need more insulin than those who are thinner. If you start to reduce your food intake you will probably have to reduce your insulin.

WARNING – Some people discover that they can control their weight just by reducing their insulin. The blood glucose levels run high, the body cannot use fuel properly and weight loss occurs. This is a dangerous step and could lead to the serious condition of ketoacidosis. It is important therefore when adjusting your food or insulin intake to check your blood glucose levels.

If you feel you need further guidance ask your doctor to refer you to a state registered dietitian. A dietitian can recommend a calorie intake and eating plan which suits your lifestyle, is medically safe and which contains the correct balance of nutrients.

Body Mass Index (BMI)

Your weight is often calculated as BMI which expresses adult weight in relation to height. From this you will be advised if you need to lose weight to help control your diabetes. Your GP will record your BMI in your notes.

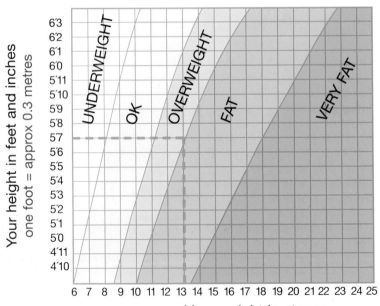

To calculate your BMI: $BMI = \dfrac{\text{weight (kg)}}{\text{height (m)}^2}$

A BMI of 20–25 is classed as a healthy weight (see the chart above). You do not need to lose weight.

A BMI of 25–30 is classed as overweight. The health risks for those in this range are associated with the extra weight being carried around your middle.

A BMI greater than 30 is associated with significantly increased health risks.

Alcohol

There is no reason why the moderate use of alcohol should not be a pleasant part of your life. However, you may want to think about what you drink and when.

Diabetes UK recommends the following maximum intake of alcohol:

2–3 units of alcohol a day for a man
1–2 units of alcohol a day for a woman

where 1 unit =
half a pint of ordinary beer, lager or cider
1 pub measure of spirits
1 glass of wine (125 ml glass)
1 small glass of sherry
1 measure of vermouth or aperitif

■ Drinking alcohol increases your likelihood of having a low blood glucose. Therefore:

1. Do not drink on an empty stomach.
2. Do not substitute alcoholic drinks for your usual meal.

■ It is important to remember that all alcoholic drinks also contain calories and should therefore be limited if you are overweight.
■ Low sugar beers are best avoided as they are higher in alcohol than normal beers.
■ Always use low calorie/sugar-free mixers and be careful of home measures.
■ Never drink and drive.

■ Summary

- ■ Eat regular meals and snacks, if needed, based on plenty of starchy carbohydrate foods eg bread, potatoes, rice, pasta and cereals.
- ■ If you are overweight try very hard to lose weight.
- ■ Watch your fat intake and avoid eating lots of fat and fatty foods.
- ■ Limit your sugar intake by restricting your intake of sweet and sugary foods and drinks.
- ■ Eat plenty of high-fibre foods, including fruit and vegetables.
- ■ Use salt in moderation.
- ■ Take care with alcohol.
- ■ Try to take regular exercise.

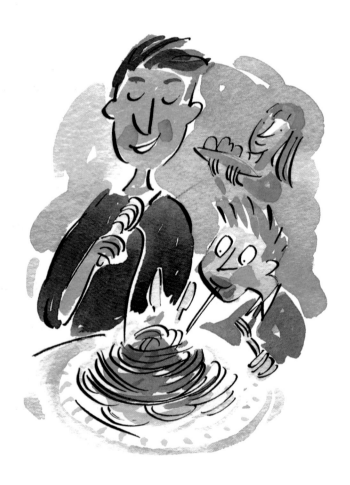

4 Is Your Treatment Effective?

The aim of treatment is to return your blood glucose level to as near normal as possible and to maintain it within acceptable limits. You will want to be sure that your insulin doses are correct. You will also want to know that the amount and type of food you eat are appropriate, ie that the balance is right. Unfortunately, how you feel is not an accurate guide to the level of your blood glucose. Symptoms of diabetes – thirst, weight loss and the passing of large amounts of urine – appear only if your diabetes is badly out of control. Even with moderately high levels of blood glucose – the sorts of levels which can, over a period of years, lead to serious complications – you may have no symptoms.

Therefore, it is essential that you make some form of check on the glucose levels in the body. You will need to repeat these checks at relatively frequent intervals.

This chapter describes how you can do these tests and when you should do them.

■ Why you need to carry out tests

The tests are necessary for three reasons:

1. To help you to understand what causes high or low blood glucose levels – this will help you make appropriate adjustments, in order to avoid these.
2. To determine if your treatment is correct – if it is not, you will be able to make changes in the type and dose of insulin, or in the size and timing of your meals.
3. To reassure yourself that the best possible control is being achieved – this will help to ensure your long-term health.

■ Blood tests versus urine tests

There are two possible ways of testing blood glucose. One is to test the blood and the other is to test the urine. Blood tests tell you exactly what is happening at the time you test. Urine is a rather more indirect method of telling you what is happening in the blood.

Urine tests are easy to perform, but have the disadvantage that they only tell you when the blood glucose has been too high and not when it is too low. They are, therefore, less informative than blood tests.

Blood tests, on the other hand, have significant advantages. They give an exact reading of the blood glucose at the time of testing. They enable you to measure your own blood glucose levels accurately, while at home, work or wherever you might be. They help you, therefore, to tell at any time if your blood glucose is too high or too low. It is easier to adjust your treatment with blood tests.

In addition, if you are unwell and need to take corrective action (see section on ketoacidosis, page 109) it is much easier and safer to work out what insulin you should be taking, based on blood rather than urine tests.

We would strongly recommend that you should if possible do blood tests. In some instances, ie very small children, or for those who feel they just cannot do blood tests (as happens sometimes during adolescence), urine tests can, however, be a useful alternative. Furthermore, there are parts of the world where blood testing equipment is unavailable. Details of urine as well as blood tests are therefore provided.

■ Blood tests

Technique

Blood tests require you to obtain a drop of blood, which must then be allowed to react with a specially prepared testing strip.

A drop of blood can be obtained by pricking the finger

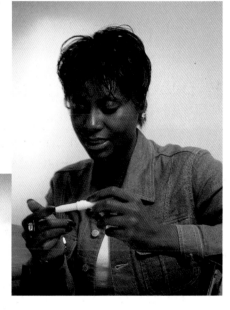

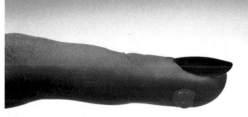

The drop of blood should be large enough to cover the test zones on the strip

Depending on the test used, the blood glucose level is determined in different ways. Some strips are designed to change colour after the blood has been applied. After wiping, the colour is compared with a chart. However, with most meters, the blood is applied to the strip and the meter reads the result automatically without wiping. However they are obtained, the results should then be recorded.

Glucose test strips

A selection of glucose test kits

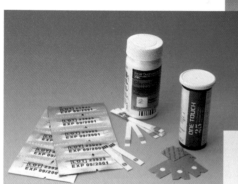

A selection of glucose test kits

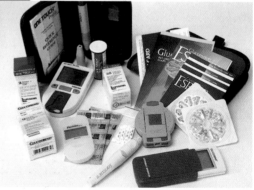

A selection of glucose meters

If you are colour blind, or have sight problems, you may not be able to read the strips by eye. In this case you will certainly need a meter. Otherwise strips read by eye are found to give results as accurate as those read by a meter. Some people, however, do not feel happy with the colour matching. In this case, do ask about the possibility of using a meter. New methods of testing the blood are being introduced all the time. If you are unhappy with the method you have been taught ask your clinic for alternatives. You can choose the method that suits you best. Remember, blood tests are simple to perform and are usually almost painless.

Recording the results

It is wise to jot down the results of the tests as soon as you do them. This may not be absolutely essential if you are using a meter with a memory. Even so, these only store a limited number of results. It is better to keep your own record. It is much easier to work out the reasons for high and low tests if you write them down at the time. Memory can play tricks. If you wish to discuss the tests with your doctor, it is much more useful if you have got some written results to look at together.

| Month | | | | | | | Test time | | | | | Insulin | | Comments |
Day	Date	Before breakfast	After breakfast	Before lunch	After lunch	Before dinner	Evening	Before bed		am	pm	Reactions, medication, illness, etc.
	1	10		7		4				28	14	
	2						10			28	14	
	3	2		4		7				28	14	
	4	7						7		28	14	
	5	7	2*							28		*Hypoglycaemic reaction at 12.30

Blood tests – recording the test results. Always record your test using a record diary such as this

Interpreting the results and making adjustments

Remember that the blood glucose level normally goes up and down. It rises after meals. It falls again 2–3 hours after meals. It is usually lowest just before meals. In people without diabetes the variation is quite small. The accepted way of expressing blood glucose concentration is in millimoles per litre. This is written as mmol/l, eg 8 mmol/l. The main point to remember is that the normal range of blood glucose before meals is between 4 and 7 mmol/l. If you are aiming for good control, try to ensure that most of your blood glucose levels remain below 10 mmol/l, even after meals. If you have trouble achieving this, some change in your routine may be necessary.

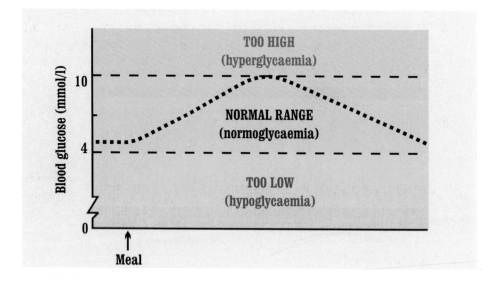

The normal range of blood glucose before and after meals

What should you do if the tests are high or low?

The aim of your treatment is to get your blood glucose as close as possible to the normal range. Your blood test will help you to achieve this. It is important that you try to get 'most' of the tests right. Because of the nature of your diabetes, it is quite likely that an occasional test will be higher or lower than ideal. Do not be alarmed by this. Odd high tests do you no harm. The aim is for your average level to be at an acceptable level. If you get the majority of your tests within this range you will be doing very well. There will, however, be times when you will need to make changes in response to high or low tests. These are discussed in detail in Chapter 5.

How often should the blood be tested?

To start with you will be asked to perform tests several times a day. This will help you to understand what causes changes in your blood glucose. Once your control is good tests may only be necessary once or twice a day. This, however, will depend on the variety of your lifestyle. If your dosage of insulin needs changing fairly frequently, more tests may be needed. However, there are certain occasions when you may find it particularly useful to carry out tests more often, eg:

- If you are troubled by low blood glucose (hypoglycaemia).
- If your work, exercise or meal times vary a great deal.
- During the week or two before a routine clinic visit. More frequent tests then will enable you and your doctor to discuss whether any changes in treatment might be needed.
- During pregnancy.
- During menstruation.
- Before or during long journeys if you are driving.

When are blood tests essential?

There are three occasions when testing is really important:

1. If you feel unwell.
2. If you suspect that your blood glucose is falling too low. This is especially important if you are about to drive, or embark on something hazardous.
3. If you are planning a pregnancy (see page 140).

Testing the average level of blood glucose

As suggested above, you will want to know whether most of the tests are falling in the acceptable range or not. If you do a lot of blood tests, you may be able to work it out yourself, but this can be quite complicated. There are now single blood tests which can do this for you. They can only be performed by a laboratory. There are two main types, one called Haemoglobin A_1 or A_1C. One blood sample provides a good estimate of the average level of blood glucose in the 6 weeks before the test.

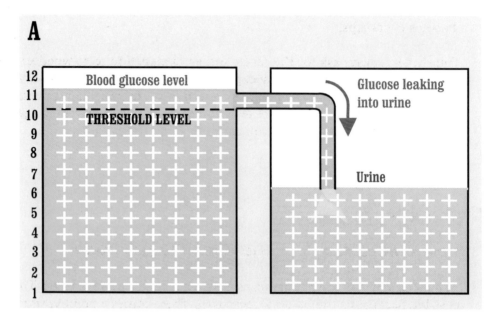

Urine test positive: The blood glucose level has exceeded the threshold level and is leaking into the urine, which means that a urine test will be positive

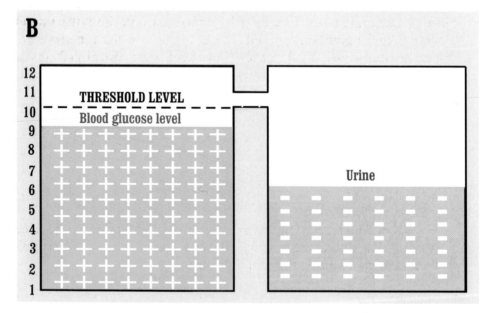

Urine test negative: The blood glucose level has not exceeded the threshold level, so none has leaked into the urine. In this case, a test will be negative

These tests will normally be performed whenever you attend for your diabetes check-ups.

You should always ask for the result and an explanation as to whether it is satisfactory. If it is within the acceptable range your treatment is working very well. If it is too high, then you may need to make some adjustments, eg you might need to do some more tests yourself, or perhaps make changes in your dosage of insulin, or what you eat.

■ Urine tests

How urine tests work and their interpretation

The blood glucose can be measured indirectly by testing your urine. This is possible because as the blood glucose rises, there comes a point at which it starts to leak into the urine. This happens when the level of the blood glucose is too high, usually above about 10 mmol/l. Therefore, if the blood glucose has been higher than this level since you last passed urine, a test for glucose in the urine will be positive. If the blood glucose has not exceeded this level (normal) the urine test will be negative. If the test is positive, the amount of glucose present gives an approximate guide to how high the level in the blood has risen above the threshold. Thus, with your type of diabetes, most tests should be negative. But, remember, urine tests are only of limited value, because they do not tell you when the blood glucose is too low.

Which urine test?

Three tests, illustrated below, are commonly available in the United Kingdom. They all involve placing a strip of special paper in the stream of urine, and then observing the colour change.

1. Diastix
2. Diabur-Test 5000
3. Ketodiastix measures both glucose and ketones; see 'Testing for ketones' on page 79.

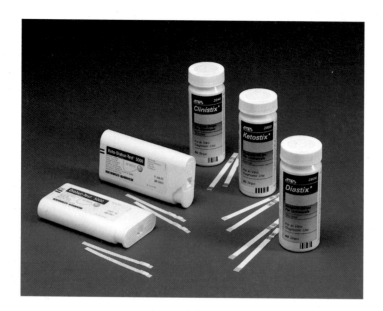

Urine test kits

Urine tests depend on a colour change, so if you cannot see well, or you are colour blind, you may not be able to detect the change, and the tests may need to be done for you.

Urine tests are easily performed. You remove the strip from its container. Insert the end with a pad on it in the stream of urine for a second or two. Tap the excess fluid off. Wait for 30 or 60 seconds, according to the instructions on the container. Compare the colour of the pad with the chart on the side of the container.

How often should you test?

To start with, you will be asked to test before each meal and last thing at night. This routine testing will help you to understand what increases your blood glucose – and therefore makes your urine tests positive – and ensures that your insulin dose is correct. As your blood glucose returns to normal, and if all your urine tests become negative, only a few tests a week may be required, just to reassure you that all is well.

There are occasions, however, when you must test several times a day:

- ■ If you feel unwell
- ■ If your overall control is poor.

When should you test?

Ideally, all tests should be negative, but it is not always possible to achieve this. Testing before a meal is preferable; testing after a meal may produce positive results, since there is usually a small peak in the blood glucose immediately after eating.

Testing for ketones

If you are having problems with very high blood glucose levels it may be recommended that you test for ketones. This may be particularly helpful if you have been admitted to hospital with ketoacidosis.

Ketones are fat breakdown products. They are produced in large quantities when you are very short of insulin. This quite often happens when you are ill. Testing will help ensure that you adjust the insulin dose and avoid ketoacidosis. The tests are performed in a similar manner to urine tests for glucose, using a dipstick.

Urine tests can be misleading

Urine tests can be misleading. For example, some people are understandably perplexed when they feel hypoglycaemic, but their urine test is positive for glucose.

This occurs because some of the urine being tested may have been formed as much as one or two hours earlier, when the blood glucose was still high. Since that time, however, the blood glucose may have returned to a low level. The earlier overspill of glucose from the blood (when the level was high) will still, however, be registering in the urine. This will give a positive result to your test. This problem may be overcome by emptying the bladder, waiting a short time (about half an hour), emptying the bladder a second time, and testing this urine specimen. This procedure, which is called 'double-voiding', produces a result which is more likely to relate to the blood glucose level at the time of testing.

Another reason for a false result is that some people leak glucose into the urine even when the blood glucose level is not increased – they have what is called 'a low renal threshold'. In such cases, testing will show the urine to be full of glucose, even though the blood glucose is normal. Clearly, to increase the insulin dose would merely cause the blood glucose to fall too low. This condition is rare, but if you think you have a low renal threshold you can check the situation by means of a blood test.

■ Watching your weight

For most people regular weighing is not necessary. It is wise to keep your weight as near normal as possible. Becoming overweight does make your diabetes control more difficult. Your weight will be checked when you attend for your check-ups. If you feel you are putting on too much weight, do keep a check yourself.

■ A final comment

You should never omit tests altogether, because without them you really have no idea what your control is like.

■ If you perform regular blood tests, it is not necessary to carry out urine tests as well.

■ If you have doubts about your control – test more often.

■ Ask for the results of your averaging test whenever you attend for a check-up.

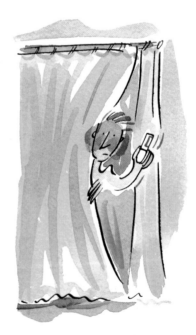

5 Keeping Good Control

This chapter describes changes you may need to make to ensure good control of your diabetes.

Your aims should be:

■ To maintain the level of your blood glucose within acceptable limits for most of the time. This is usually between 4 and 7 mmol/l.
■ To ensure freedom from hypoglycaemia.
■ To carry on life as you would wish.

These goals are more easily achieved by some people than by others. Some individuals have a way of life that may vary considerably from one day to the next. They may, therefore, need some variation in the amount of insulin injected, or in the type and amount of food eaten.

■ Should you make changes yourself?

Many people are concerned about making changes in their treatment on their own. You may feel that it is up to your doctor or nurse specialist to tell you when to make changes. This is especially likely in the early stages of your treatment.

However, your lifestyle will never be quite the same as anybody else's. Although the professionals can and will give you general advice, you will need to learn to make adjustments yourself.

You need not worry that you will do yourself harm by making the sorts of adjustments that are advised below. You will certainly feel happier if you are in complete control. The initial stages of your treatment are, in part, trial and error. You will, however, come to absolutely no harm during this period while you learn which adjustments are successful or unsuccessful.

■ When should you make adjustments?

You should consider whether you need to change your insulin or food if:

■ You are having frequent hypoglycaemic reactions.

■ Your blood tests are regularly higher than 8 mmol/l (or your urine tests show glucose consistently).

■ The blood test performed to give an overall estimate for the previous six weeks is running high.

■ The amount of physical exercise you take varies considerably from day to day.

Action now or action later?

There are some occasions where it is essential to make changes straight away.

■ If you are feeling unwell, especially if you are being sick, you are likely to need a change in your dose of insulin. Your blood glucose will usually rise and it is important to increase the dose and/or frequency of insulin.

■ If you are suffering from a low blood glucose level (hypoglycaemia) you must put this right straight away. (See Chapter 7.)

Both these situations are dealt with in detail in Chapter 6.

For those with a fairly regular lifestyle, and for those on two injections of insulin a day, it is probably best to:

1. Avoid changing your insulin dose on the basis of a single test. If, however, repeated tests indicate a definite pattern of highs or lows, then make changes.

2. Remember that tests in general tell you only how well the previous injection of insulin has worked.

Those with a more varied lifestyle, and especially those requiring more than two injections a day, may need to make adjustments more frequently and in a different way.

Rather than looking back at trends, you may wish to react immediately to individual tests, making adjustments to cope with the next period of the day.

■ What types of adjustments might be necessary?

Various adjustments are possible:

- ■ Changing your dose of insulin
- ■ Changing the type of insulin and/or the balance between quick- and slow-acting insulins
- ■ Changing the timing of your insulin injections
- ■ Changing the amount, or type, of food you eat
- ■ Increasing the number of injections
- ■ Altering your injection sites.

Adjustments with twice-daily insulin

Changing your dose of insulin

Depending on the results of your tests, you might find it necessary to modify your dose of insulin. For example:

- ■ If all your tests, morning and evening, are high, you need more insulin.

- ■ If all your morning tests are high and the remainder normal, you may need more insulin in the evening. But, be careful – sometimes the blood glucose may fall very low during the night, then rise before breakfast, when the insulin level has dropped. An increase in insulin may make this worse. Changing the timing of the evening injection or the type of insulin to a longer-acting one may be needed.

Blood									Urine			
Before breakfast	2 hours after breakfast	Before midday meal	2 hours after midday meal	Before evening meal	2 hours after evening meal	Before bed	During night		Before breakfast	Before midday meal	Before evening meal	Before bed
13		7		7		10			++	neg	neg	neg
15	4	7		7		7			++++	neg	neg	neg
17	4	7		7		4			++++	neg	neg	neg

High morning tests. These results suggest the need for a larger dose of insulin in the evening

■ If you have regular hypoglycaemic reactions in the late morning a reduction in the morning dose of quick- or short-acting insulin may be appropriate. (Similarly, the evening dose may need reducing if you have had a reaction after your evening meal before bedtime.) Consider other possibilities: did you have a mid-morning snack or an adequate breakfast?

Changing the type of insulin and/or the balance between insulins

As indicated in a previous chapter, there are a variety of insulins, very quick-, quick- or slow-acting. The duration of action of an insulin injection may be increased by increasing the dose. This can result in too high a level of insulin shortly after the insulin injection. For example:

■ Suppose you are taking insulin twice a day and all your midday tests are normal, or slightly low, but at 5.00 or 6.00 pm your tests are too high. Then your insulin is acting quickly, but not lasting for long enough. Perhaps you need a mixture of quick- and slow-acting insulins. If you are already taking such a mixture, a decrease in the quick, and an increase in the slow, may be appropriate.

Blood									Urine			
Before breakfast	2 hours after breakfast	Before midday meal	2 hours after midday meal	Before evening meal	2 hours after evening meal	Before bed	During night		Before breakfast	Before midday meal	Before evening meal	Before bed
7		4		13		7			neg	neg	++	neg
4	7	2		17		4			neg	neg	++++	neg
7		4		15		7			neg	neg	++++	neg

High evening tests. These results suggest the need for a change in the type and/or dose of insulin

■ In contrast, if your tests at midday are high and your pre-evening meal tests normal, perhaps more quick-acting clear insulin is needed in the morning.

Blood									Urine			
Before breakfast	2 hours after breakfast	Before midday meal	2 hours after midday meal	Before evening meal	2 hours after evening meal	Before bed	During night		Before breakfast	Before midday meal	Before evening meal	Before bed
4	15	13		7		7			neg	++	neg	neg
7		15		7	4	7			neg	++++	neg	neg
7		13		4		7			neg	++++	neg	neg

High midday tests and normal evening tests. These results suggest the need for more quick-acting clear insulin in the morning

■ Similar principles apply to the evening injection. If your pre-bedtime test is low, but your early morning test is high, you need less quick-acting insulin and more slow-acting insulin before your main evening meal.

Changing the timing of your insulin injection

When using quick-acting or a mixture of quick- and slow-acting insulins, it is usually necessary to have a reasonable gap between the injection and the meal. We usually recommend half an hour, to allow the insulin to get into the blood stream. This allows the increasing level of insulin to cope with the glucose rise that occurs after a meal. If you find your tests are going very high one to two hours after a meal, then you may improve this by increasing the time between the injection and the meal. Very quick-acting insulins are given immediately before or as you start eating. This is obviously more convenient but these insulins do not suit everybody as they sometimes do not last long enough.

Changing meal times

Undoubtedly there will be times when you want to change the timing of your meals.

Late evening meal

When you eat later than usual, simply have a small snack at the time you would normally eat your evening meal (to balance any insulin that might be left over from your previous dose), then inject your insulin before your main meal as usual.

If you intend eating an evening meal very much later than normal, ie 2 to 3 hours, then you should have slightly less insulin before your meal, otherwise the effects could continue into the next morning. If in doubt about the time at which you will be eating, assume that the meal will be late. Have a small snack in the meantime.

Late breakfast

Occasionally you may choose to have a lie-in and a late breakfast. This is perfectly acceptable, but it is best not to delay your breakfast by more than two hours. Have your insulin before your late breakfast. However, you may find you need a cup of tea or a biscuit at your normal breakfast time. This may be necessary because there is some insulin left over from the night before. Otherwise your blood glucose may go too low.

Working shifts

When working shifts, especially if the shifts change from day to day or week to week, your meal times are likely to be different. You will need to vary the time at which you inject your insulin. The timing of injections will certainly be different on working and rest days. These changes are possible with twice-daily insulin, but are much easier if you use more injections of quick- or very quick-acting insulin (see Chapter 6).

Adjusting for exercise

If you take regular exercise or perform heavy work at regular times of the day or week, it is worth considering reducing your insulin dose to allow for this.

If the times at which you are likely to do this are unpredictable, then you may prefer to take more to eat just beforehand.

Sometimes exercise may have a delayed effect. In particular, 'heavy training' type of exercise may cause hypoglycaemia up to 24 hours later.

Changing the amount of food you eat

As indicated in a previous chapter, the food that you eat and the insulin that you use have to be balanced. Changes may be necessary in what you eat. For example:

- If your tests are running high, this may be because you are eating more than usual. This is more likely to happen if you are taking refined sugar (sucrose) (see Chapter 3). Cutting down the size of your meals, and in particular any refined sugar, may help.

- If your weight is normal, and yet you are still hungry (or losing weight), there is no harm in increasing the size of your meals. Try to keep this increase fairly consistent from one day to the next – decide at which meals you are going to eat more and try to keep those meals to a similar size from one day to the next. If your tests begin to show high blood glucose levels, then an increase in insulin dosage should easily correct this.

■ If you feel slightly 'hypo' at around noon to one o'clock an extra snack mid-morning, or an earlier midday meal, often solves the problem. This may be easier than reducing your dose of insulin.

	Blood									Urine			
Before breakfast	2 hours after breakfast	Before midday meal	2 hours after midday meal	Before evening meal	2 hours after evening meal	Before bed	During night		Before breakfast	Before midday meal	Before evening meal	Before bed	
7		2		7		4							
4		2		4		7							
7		2*		7		7							

Comments: reaction at 12.30

Low midday tests. These results suggest the need for a mid-morning snack or an earlier midday meal

■ As a general rule, whenever your blood tests indicate that your blood glucose is too low, you should have something to eat, even if you have no symptoms.

Temporary changes in insulin dosage

The adjustments to your insulin dosage that are necessary when you are ill are described in Chapter 7 (page 110). Often you may find that minor illnesses, such as colds, cause your blood glucose level to rise for a few days. Women may find that their menstrual periods cause an increase, or decrease, in blood glucose level. This variation may precede the actual period by a couple of days. Temporary changes in your work pattern, or the amount of physical exercise you take, may also require short-term changes.

The commonest cause of fluctuations in your blood glucose is probably emotional stress. You may find that the only indication that you are under pressure will be a raised blood glucose. If you are sure that this 'high' is not an isolated result, you can respond to it by increasing your insulin. You may then be able to reduce it after a few days when the tests return to normal.

Increasing the number of injections

You may find that, despite alterations of the kind described above, you are still having difficulties with control. It may be that the timing of injections and/or meals is too rigid for you. Your lifestyle may be too variable and you may not feel in control with only two injections a day.

You might consider increasing the number of injections of quick-acting insulin. This could be only temporary. If, for example, you are unwell, one or two extra injections of quick-acting insulin may be needed just to keep control for a day or two.

Alternatively, you might find a system with more frequent injections of quick-acting insulin before each meal and slow-acting insulin at bedtime suits your needs better. The advantages and details of this are described in Chapter 6.

A single increase from two to three injections a day may be the solution for those having difficulty with overnight control. Quite often people find their early morning tests are high. If, however, they increase the dose of insulin before their evening meal they have a hypoglycaemic reaction during the early hours of the morning. An easy remedy is to have some quick- or very quick-acting insulin alone before the evening meal and then a third injection of longer-acting insulin before bedtime. This also allows more flexibility of timing and size of your evening meal. Misjudgment of the dose of pre-evening meal insulin can easily be detected at the bedtime test. The bedtime dose of slower-acting insulin can then be adjusted.

Altering your injection site

You may find differences in your glucose control when you inject in different sites. Generally speaking, the insulin is absorbed more quickly when injected into the abdomen than into the leg. It is best to use a large area. However, there is plenty of space within say, a thigh, or the abdominal area, to move the injections around. If you do find differences between injections in the abdomen or thigh, then we suggest you choose one area for the morning, and one for the evening injection. Since quicker action may be needed in the morning consider the abdomen for the morning injection. In contrast, since you need the injection to last longer to cover the night – use the thigh. This will provide more consistency.

Remember that if you continue to inject in *exactly* the same site all the time, ie an area of say a fifty pence piece, you will run into problems. The tissue will form a sort of scar or a large fatty lump. This will not only be unsightly but also interfere with the absorption of insulin.

■ Summary

- ■ Do not be afraid of making changes.
- ■ Provided you check your tests and see what happens you are unlikely to come to any harm.
- ■ When making changes for the first time, test regularly to see if they work.
- ■ Very small changes are likely to be of little benefit.
- ■ Frequent chopping and changing may be confusing. It is better to make changes and then observe what happens over the next few days. If things are not right try something different.
- ■ If in doubt about the changes you should ring your diabetes doctor or nurse specialist.
- ■ Not everybody has to make changes. If your tests are good, and you are happy, carry on as you are.

Finally, if you are unhappy with your control or with the restrictions on your life because of your diabetes, consider the more flexible system with multiple injections described in the next chapter.

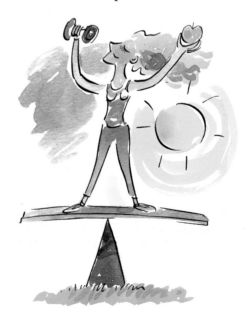

6 Multiple Injection Treatment and the Use of Insulin Pumps

The sorts of adjustments that can be made using two injections a day were described in the previous chapter. You may have decided that this does not give you the sort of control that you want. Alternatively, you may feel that it is too restrictive in terms of when and what you eat. You may have difficulties in adapting to variation in the amount of physical exercise you take. This chapter describes the use of multiple injections, the flexibility they provide ·and details of how you might adopt this regimen yourself. Finally, the use of insulin pumps as an alternative to standard syringes is described.

■ The advantages of increasing the number of injections

It is worth at this stage looking back at our description on pages 12–13 of how the normal pancreas works. The pancreas responds to each meal by releasing insulin in proportion to the rise of blood glucose after a meal, ie the pancreas is able to calculate the dose of insulin required for each meal. This ensures that the blood glucose only rises slightly after each meal and then returns fairly quickly to normal. When not eating, for example overnight, there is normally a steady trickle of insulin from the pancreas. This compensates for the steady trickle of glucose into the blood stream (from the liver), and keeps the blood glucose steady.

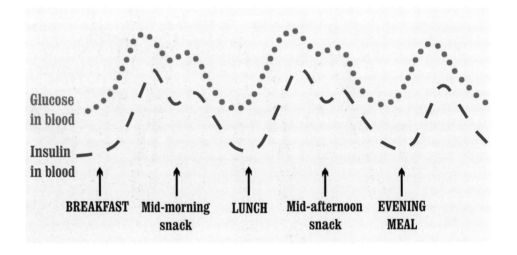

Glucose in blood

Insulin in blood

**BREAKFAST   Mid-morning   LUNCH   Mid-afternoon   EVENING
                    snack   snack   MEAL**

Insulin levels keep closely in step with glucose levels throughout the day

The purpose of insulin treatment is to try to copy the normal pancreas as much as possible. This may be difficult with only two injections a day. Even when using mixtures of quick- and slow-acting insulin, this system may not be sensitive enough to control the changes in your blood glucose.

Your meals are bound to vary in size and content. Even when paying very close attention to when and what you eat, you may find that your blood glucose goes unexpectedly high or low on occasion.

You may want to make major changes in the size and/or type of meals you eat on different days, holidays, birthdays, etc, or delay meals for the sake of convenience. Adjusting twice-daily insulin injections may not cope with this. Your physical activity may vary rather more than you might predict. Very variable work patterns, shift working and intense physical training can lead to difficulties with control.

These situations can more easily be coped with using a multiple injection system.

With the new pen devices frequent injections of insulin can be given very easily. It is simpler to carry around insulin in a pen device than standard syringes and bottles.

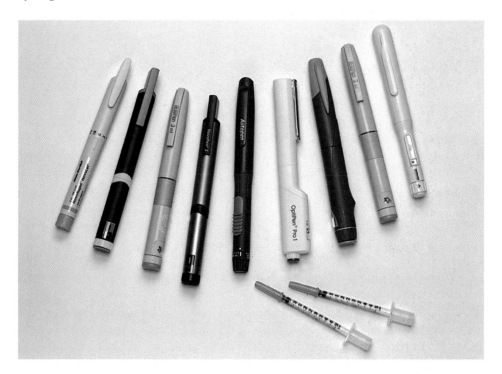

A selection of pen devices

The advantages of multiple injections, therefore, are:

- First and most important, they give you more overall control of your life and your diabetes.
- They will provide you with greater flexibility in the timing and content of your meals.
- They allow better adjustment for heavy exercise, shift working, variable work patterns, etc.
- They allow you greater flexibility in your social life.
- They may prevent the problems of night-time hypos and early morning high blood glucose.

■ How to use multiple injections

Frequency of injections

The aim is to provide a surge of insulin before each of your main meals, with a background level throughout the 24 hours. For most people this means a quick-acting insulin before breakfast, lunch and evening meal and a slow-acting one at bedtime.

It is not always necessary to have three injections of quick-acting insulin. Some people may find that an injection before breakfast, and an injection before the evening meal, with a trickle of background insulin given just before bedtime, works well. Others with very variable meal patterns may find that more than three injections of quick-acting insulin work better.

Some background insulin is needed. This is usually given last thing at night. Sometimes, however, this does not provide enough of the trickle of insulin between meals during the daytime. For these people additional slow-acting insulin may be required with the first injection of quick-acting before breakfast.

Adjusting the dose of insulin

The chief advantage of multiple injection systems is that they allow easy adjustments in the dosage of insulin to cope with changes in your meal size, or type, and the amount of exercise you take. The intention, therefore, is to provide bigger doses of insulin for large meals and smaller doses for small meals.

Let us assume that you wish to have a large meal, perhaps with a sweet dessert. You will need to work out the effect such a meal will have on your glucose and the dose of insulin which will keep the blood glucose level roughly within the normal range. You can find out for yourself, by testing before a meal and, say, an hour to two hours later with a certain dose of insulin. If you find the blood glucose goes very high, then you will need to increase the dose of insulin when you have such a meal again.

In contrast, you may decide that you want to skip a meal, or have a much smaller meal. You will then need to reduce the dose of insulin just before it, or possibly, if you have no meal at all, miss out the dose altogether. This last step only works if there is some background insulin. See what happens when you miss a meal by taking some tests. If the blood glucose starts rising when this happens, it is probably more sensible to have a much smaller dose of insulin rather than omitting it altogether.

■ Calculating doses

At this stage many people may be asking whether there are simple formulae to calculate the exact doses of insulin for meals of particular size or content. Such calculations have been worked out, but in practice they do not work particularly well. This is because everybody is different. The rate of absorption of food and the speed at which insulin is absorbed from the injection site vary from person to person. Therefore, two people eating identical foods at identical times may require quite different doses of insulin. It is necessary, therefore, for you to work out for yourself exactly what your insulin needs are. This means that, in the learning stage, you will need to take quite frequent tests, and establish for yourself the ideal dosages of insulin in relation to the timing of your meals, exercise, etc.

Most people require about one-third of their total daily insulin dose as the slow-acting trickle, and two-thirds divided between the meals in the quick-acting injection. A larger dose of quick-acting is often needed before breakfast than before lunch, even though breakfast may be a smaller meal. The reasons for this are not entirely understood. Since most busy people have their largest meal in the evening a larger dose may be needed for this meal.

Quick- or very quick-acting insulin?

With the introduction of very quick-acting insulins, many people find these much more convenient, especially when using multiple injections. They do not, indeed should not, be given 30 minutes before a meal, but immediately before or just as you start eating.

However, their effect does not usually last as long as that of ordinary quick-acting insulins, ie an injection before breakfast at 7.30 am may not last until lunch at 1.00 pm.

Very quick-acting insulins before the evening meal do have the advantage that their effect has usually worn off completely before bedtime. There is little risk of overlap with slow-acting insulin given at evening meal or bedtime. The risk of low blood sugar – hypoglycaemic reactions – during the night are greatly reduced.

Although you will need to work out a system that suits you personally, here are some examples which may help you decide the sorts of variations that will satisfy your needs

■ Case history 1

Coping with variable meals and work

Bob is a 35-year-old travelling sales-man. He has been taking a twice-daily mixture of quick- and slow-acting insulin before his break-fast and before his evening meal. He finds, because of his work, that he has difficulty having his meals on time. If he delays them, however, he goes 'hypo'. He wants to switch to the multiple injection regime. Up until now his total dose has been around 40 units, 26 units in the morning and 14 units in the evening.

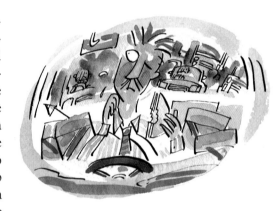

He has been advised to take quick-acting insulin, 10 units before his break-fast, 6 units before his midday meal, and 6 units before his evening meal, and 10 units of slow-acting insulin before he goes to bed.

Comment

You will note that Bob was advised to take a higher dose before his breakfast as opposed to his lunch or evening meal.

You may also have noted that his total daily dose is less than that which he was taking previously. This is because, using multiple injections, rather less insulin is required than with twice-daily injections.

Bob started this treatment and did quite a lot of tests. These are shown in the chart.

You will see that Bob has been doing tests both before and after meals. This may seem like a nuisance but it is the only way to work out whether the dose of insulin is appropriate for the size of meals that he is having.

On the Wednesday, his blood glucose went rather high after his midday meal (marked *). On this day, instead of having his normal sandwiches and apple, he had a working lunch with steak and kidney pie, potatoes and vegetable, and a dessert. He was advised to take 4 extra units for such a meal. The next day he had a similar meal again, and with the extra units of insulin, he kept good control. On Friday, because of his work, he was unable to get his lunch. He sensibly checked, at his normal lunch-time, to make sure he was not going too low. He found his blood glucose was 7, so that was all right. Therefore he omitted his insulin. He re-checked his blood two hours later. He found it was 8. That was at three in the afternoon. When he checked again before his evening meal time, around 6.30 pm, he found that it had gone up to 15.

Bob's test results	Breakfast Before	Breakfast After	Lunch Before	Lunch After	Evening meal Before	Evening meal After	Bedtime
Monday Blood glucose	5	9	4	8	5	10	7
Insulin dose	(10)		(6)		(6)		[10]
Tuesday Blood glucose	3		6	10	4		8
Insulin dose	(10)		(6)		(6)		[10]
Wednesday Blood glucose	7		8	15*	12		12
Insulin dose	(10)		(6)		(6)		[10]
Thursday Blood glucose	6	10	7	10		10	6
Insulin dose	(10)		(10)		(6)		[10]
Friday Blood glucose	3		7	10	15	19	13
Insulin dose	(10)		—		(6)		[10]

Switching from two to four injections (three quick-acting (◯)and one slow (▢). Effect of a large lunch (Wednesday), correction on Thursday and effect of omitting insulin on Friday.

You will note that Bob was able, quite safely, to omit his midday dose. The effect of his morning insulin, taken before his breakfast, had worn off, so he was not at risk of hypoglycaemia. However, the morning insulin did not last through to the evening, so by his evening mealtime his blood glucose was running quite high as he had not had a midday dose.

The next time that this happened he would be advised not to omit the insulin altogether, but to have a smaller dose, say 2 units, at around the time when he would have eaten, just to retain overall control.

■ Case history 2

Night working

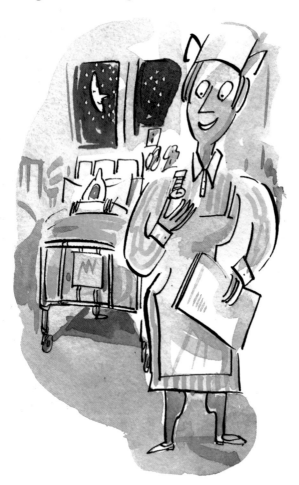

Jane is a nurse and, for the first time, she has been asked to do night-duty. She is already taking multiple injections.

The day that she starts night-duty, her shift will start at 9 o'clock in the evening and she will work through to the following morning, and she would be expected to go to bed during the next day, prior to the next night-shift.

Jane's test results for changing shifts

MONDAY							
Time	0800		1300		1800	2100	2400
Meals	Breakfast		Lunch		Evening Meal	Start Shift	Meal
Insulin: Quick-acting	12		6		14	—	6
Slow-acting	—		—		—	—	—

TUESDAY								
Time	0400	0800	0930		1600	1730	2100	2400
Meals	Snack	End Shift	Breakfast	Sleep		Meal	Start Shift	
Insulin: Quick-acting	4	—	—	—	—	14	—	6
Slow-acting	—	—	12	—	—	—	—	—

On the day before her night-shift (Monday, see chart) she will almost certainly not go to bed, so she will have her normal dosages of quick-acting insulin for breakfast, lunch and her evening meal before starting work. However, she would be advised not to take her normal long-acting insulin that night. Instead, because she will have a meal during the night, she can take a small dose of insulin again before this meal (6 units).

She will probably have a snack at about four in the morning and can have another small injection (4 units) before this meal, and then an injection of slow-acting insulin before her breakfast when she goes to bed during the next day.

On waking, the following evening, she can treat this as her normal 'day', ie have short-acting insulin when she has a meal when she gets up, and with her additional meals during the night.

■ Case history 3

Difficulties with control

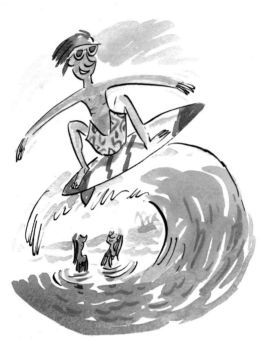

Ed is 18 years old. He has just left school and is enjoying his summer holiday. He is taking short-acting insulin before each meal, 16 units before breakfast, 12 units before lunch, and 14 units before his evening meal, with 20 units of slow-acting insulin last thing at night.

His blood sugar tests show the following:

Blood										Urine			
Before breakfast	2 hours after breakfast	Before midday meal	2 hours after midday meal	Before evening meal	2 hours after evening meal	Before bed	During night			Before breakfast	Before midday meal	Before evening meal	Before bed
13		14		18		20							

Comment

You will notice that these results are all quite high. Ed was advised to increase the dosages of short-acting insulin, as he seems to be eating quite a lot. He put all the doses of quick-acting insulin up by 2 units (to 18 units, 14 units, and 16 units, respectively) – and the slow-acting by 4 units. After this, he found that he got occasional reactions, both late morning and late afternoon. He therefore went back to his original dose. His glucose tests went high again. He was advised, therefore, to take some slow-acting insulin first thing in the morning to give a better level of background insulin. This seemed to do the trick, so that now his glucose tests returned mostly to normal.

Saturday nights

Ed is going to a big family party on Saturday night. He knows what time the meal will be. He plans to take an extra 4 units with his evening dose; this seems to work well.

The next week he is going out on Saturday night with his friends. He is not quite sure what they are going to do, or when they are going to eat. What should he do? If he takes the increased dose, and then does not get as much food as he expects, he may go 'hypo'. This will be aggravated further if he is drinking alcohol.

The best solution would be to have a smaller dose of insulin early in the evening, say 6 units and a snack, and then have no further insulin until he gets home at night. If he eats a lot more than he anticipated, his blood glucose may go up, in which case he can increase his bedtime insulin by 4 units or so to cope with this.

Staying out late

Ed may be going out, perhaps to the cinema, then having a meal at 10 or 11 o'clock. He can do as before and have a snack before he goes, with a small dose of insulin, say 4 or 6 units. He should take his pen with him and then, just before his hamburger and chips at 10.00–10.30 pm, give himself a further 6 units.

He may find that this does the trick but that, when he gets home at 2 am, his blood glucose is quite low at 4. He would be advised to halve the dose of long-acting insulin that night.

The following morning he may find that his blood glucose has risen slightly. If this just happens on an odd occasion, it is nothing to worry about. He can always give himself a bit more quick-acting insulin before breakfast, just to catch up.

■ Case history 4

Starting a new or different job

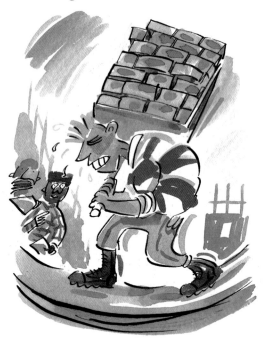

Richard is 20. He has had diabetes for several years using twice-daily insulin, and has had reasonable control. He has been unemployed for several months, but has just been offered a place as a trainee bricklayer. This will involve working on-site four days a week with day-release for training at the local college for one day. He has previously not taken a great deal of exercise.

He is worried that the increased work on a building site may cause him to go hypoglycaemic. He will obviously take considerably less physical exercise during the day at college.

He was advised to try the multiple injection system, having smaller injections of quick-acting insulin before each meal. He is going to take a packed lunch with him, so he will use his pen just before he has that.

His previous daily dose was 56 units, so the dosages he might try are: 12 units of quick-acting insulin before breakfast, 6 units before his packed lunch, and 12 units before his fairly large evening meal, and finally 16 units of slow-acting insulin at night.

Doing tests is obviously difficult while he is on the site, and he is advised just to watch out for the symptoms of hypoglycaemia, and check himself in the morning and evening. These results are good. On the day at college, he will probably require an extra couple of units at each mealtime to cope with the reduced activity. If he takes tests, he may find that he actually needs more than this, and he can make the necessary adjustments.

■ Case history 5

Intense physical activity

A well known professional footballer has had diabetes for several years and has found that the pen regimen suits him ideally.

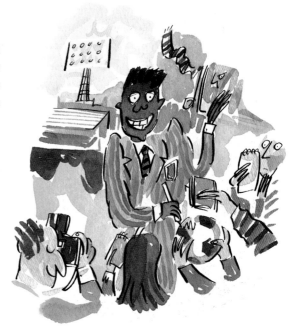

Roughly speaking his programme consists of:

- ■ Fairly intensive training, lasting an hour or two for most mornings during the week.

- ■ On Saturday, he plays a full 90 minutes.

- ■ For occasional cup games, he has to allow for the fact that they might play extra time!

- ■ There are quite frequently mid-week evening games.

He manages his insulin as follows.

He uses a pen regimen with dosage before each meal. On Saturday match days he will have his normal pre-breakfast dose. He will then have a large carbohydrate meal at between 12 noon and 1 o'clock. This meal will be considerably larger than his usual weekday meal but is of course going to be followed by some very hard physical work. He takes half his normal dose of insulin with this large carbohydrate meal. He then checks his blood glucose again after the game (and maybe at half-time) and if it is low, tops himself up with more carbohydrate.

Prior to his evening meal, he reduces this dose by 2 to 4 units because he has found that, after excessive exercise in the afternoon, he may develop hypoglycaemia later on in the evening. He checks his blood glucose again before going to bed and gives his normal overnight insulin.

On the days that he is training, during the week, he cuts his morning pre-breakfast dose by 3 to 4 units, checks his blood glucose at midday, and has a sizeable midday meal. Again he has less insulin at midday on those days. On a rest day he will have 2 to 3 units more at midday. For evening games, he cuts his pre-evening meal dose down by 3 to 4 units. He has a larger carbohydrate meal again an hour or so before the game. To avoid late hypoglycaemia in the early hours of the morning he checks his blood glucose before going to bed. If it is lowish, he cuts down his evening overnight insulin by 2 or 3 units.

■ Insulin pump therapy

The principles of using an insulin pump are identical to those of multiple injections with pen or standard syringe. The main difference is the way the insulin is delivered. However, in addition, modern pumps are designed not only to enable you to give shots of insulin before each meal or snack but also to deliver a slow trickle of 'background' insulin between meals or overnight. However, the quantity of background insulin required to control the blood sugar during these periods varies not only from person to person but also at different times throughout the day and night, ie less may be required between bedtime and 3.00 am than between 5.00 and 8.00 am or during the daytime. The pumps are designed to alter these rates automatically.

How pumps work

The pump itself is quite small and light – about the size of a cigarette packet. It delivers the insulin through a fine plastic tube connected to a specially designed fine needle which is inserted under the skin of the abdomen. The needle is slightly flexible and once inserted usually causes no discomfort.

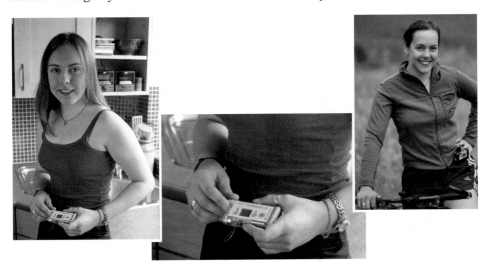

The pump is designed to give

■ Shots of insulin to cover meals and snacks whenever you require it. This is done by setting the amount of insulin you decide you need for particular meals and snacks, and then delivering it immediately using the buttons on the pump.

■ Delivering a trickle of background insulin to maintain control throughout the 24 hours. The pump can be programmed to alter this rate automatically to allow for your particular pattern of variation of need for this background insulin.

Practical aspects

■ The needle must be removed and inserted in a slightly different position every three days. If not, the point at which it is inserted may become inflamed and the delivery of insulin may be inaccurate.

■ Different lengths of tubing are available to allow full movement, ie continued use during strenuous exercise, sport, etc.

■ Wearing the pump: because the pump is small it can easily be worn without it showing: in a pocket, tucked into a bra or placed in a case

worn on a belt. During the night, using the long tubing the pump
can be placed on a bedside table, under a pillow or alternatively
there are specially designed 'sleep shorts' with a pocket.

■ Pumps must not be submerged in water. When in the bath or shower,
use of the long tubing or a shower cover means the pump can be
kept dry. Covers have been developed to allow you to swim with the
pump.

You may need to disconnect for short periods and quick-release mechanisms
are available but see warning below.

Safety

The pumps are fitted with alarms to warn you should the tubing kink,
become disconnected, or become blocked, or should the pump fail, but ...

Warning No mechanical device is 100 per cent perfect!

If the pump fails and the trickle of insulin stops you can become short of
insulin very quickly. It is different from standard injections in this respect.
With ordinary injections there is a reservoir of insulin at the site of the
injection that is relatively slowly absorbed over several hours. With the pump
the trickle is very slow and absorbed immediately. There is no reservoir.
Within half an hour or so, or possibly less, as soon as the pump stops, the
level of insulin in the blood drops to zero.

There is a risk, therefore, that you could develop the dangerous condition of
ketoacidosis quite quickly if you do not notice. Although this risk is small
you do have to be careful.

Remember, the pump is not measuring the blood sugar. You have to drive
it. You will need to decide on the amounts of insulin to be used in exactly
the same way as with multiple injections. Regular testing is essential.

Training

You will appreciate from the above that using a pump is more complicated
than using standard injections. In order to achieve success, careful training

is required. You will need to work out the amounts of insulin you personally need to cope with meals and snacks of different sizes and the changes in background insulin at different times of the day, to be programmed into your pump. And, of course, you will need to be familiar with all the practical details, connections, replacing the needle and the warning devices. This takes several days.

Multiple injections or pump?

Firstly you need to decide which method you might prefer. Secondly you will need to discuss this with your doctor or specialist nurse, who may be able to advise which might best help deal with your particular problems. There is finally a problem of cost. Pumps are expensive and at present their costs are not covered by NHS provisions. Some clinics do have some funding from charitable sources but this is generally limited.

■ Fine tuning with multiple injections and pumps – more about carbohydrate (DAFNE approach)

Whether using multiple injections or pumps, one of the difficulties is calculating the amount of insulin required for each meal or snack. There is so much variation between different meals and different foods, and this can lead to unexpectedly high or even low levels of blood sugar after meals. It is very often quite difficult to estimate how much insulin you need to inject before meals. If you are having these problems, it may be possible to adjust your insulin dose more accurately by estimating in more detail how much carbohydrate you are going to eat using the carbohydrate portion estimate.

One carbohydrate portion contains 10–12 grams of carbohydrate, 13–17 grams of carbohydrate equals 1½ carbohydrate portions and 18–22 grams of carbohydrate equals 2 carbohydrate portions. Extensive lists of the carbohydrate content of different foods are available. However, as indicated in Chapter 3, carbohydrate foods push the sugar up and down to a greater or lesser extent dependent not only on the actual total count of carbohydrate (indicated on the label in grams) but also on the types of carbohydrate and the other foods with which they are combined. We hardly ever eat pure carbohydrate. We are learning more and more about the response of the blood sugar to different carbohydrate-containing foods in meals, defined by the glycaemic index (see Chapter 3). Combining both the carbohydrate portion system and some knowledge of glycaemic index, it is possible to make more accurate estimates of the insulin required per meal.

Having decided what you want to eat (ie how many carbohydrate portions) you inject the right amount of insulin to match this. The actual amount varies from person to person depending on your usual dose, your weight and the amount of physical exercise you take. However, training programmes which are now becoming available, known as DAFNE programmes (Dose Adjustment for Normal Eating), enable you to learn much more about carbohydrate portions, glycaemic index and how to calculate how much insulin you need for each carbohydrate portion. This, of course, will need still to be combined with trial and error but may lead to much better overall control. Perhaps, more importantly, it will enable you to vary the food you eat with much more confidence that you can still avoid high and low blood sugars since the insulin dosage is more finely tuned to each meal.

■ Summary

These examples show how multiple injections can be used to give good control in a variety of circumstances. Your situation may not fit any of these exactly. However, you can see that almost any situation can be dealt with. By discussion with your diabetes specialist, or specialist nurse, it is hoped that you can develop a management regimen which not only gives good glucose control, but also allows you to do everything you want.

7 What Can Go Wrong?

This chapter looks at two important problems that can develop during treatment of your diabetes and considers how to overcome them:

1. An increase in your blood glucose due to other illnesses – this can cause some resistance to the action of insulin, and ketoacidosis.
2. Hypoglycaemia (a 'hypo' or 'reaction') – a blood glucose level which is too low, due to an imbalance between food and insulin.

It is ESSENTIAL that you are PREPARED for these problems and that you are able to deal with them. Therefore, it is important that you read and become familiar with this section of the book.

■ Ketoacidosis or severe lack of insulin

When is severe lack of insulin likely to occur?

It is most likely to happen:

■ If the dose of insulin is reduced or not given at all.
■ In the presence of illness, which increases blood glucose and ketones which cause resistance to the action of insulin.

You may think that, because you feel unwell and do not want to eat, you should reduce or even stop your insulin. This is a passport to disaster. In the absence of sufficient insulin, and especially if you are ill, your body continues to make glucose. Even if you are not eating, your blood glucose is likely to rise rather than fall as the body makes glucose in response to the illness. In addition your fat stores will be used as an alternative fuel. This results in release of fat breakdown products called ketones into the blood stream. Eventually, if untreated, these ketones will cause a diabetic coma (ketosis or ketoacidosis). This, however, will not occur if you are eating and drinking normally and can be prevented by taking the right steps. In particular, never reduce or stop your insulin.

Fortunately, symptoms develop relatively slowly (as compared with symptoms of hypoglycaemia). Diabetic coma will normally be preceded by a period of at least several hours during which time the following symptoms may occur:

- A period of thirst
- Frequent passage of urine
- Weakness
- Vomiting.

If you are using a pump and it stops for any reason, then these symptoms may develop more rapidly.

What should you do if you are unwell?

To deal effectively with your diabetes during an illness, you must BE PREPARED. If you live alone, it is a good idea to make sure that a relative, friend or neighbour knows that you are not well. It is unlikely that you will feel like reading this book when you are unwell, so get the following steps clear in your mind beforehand.

If you lose your appetite, feel sick or are vomiting, you should take the following steps:

STEP 1 – take fluids

You should try to have regular amounts of fluids containing sugar. This is because fluids are absorbed from the stomach in considerable amounts even when you are vomiting. They are usually kept down long enough for absorption to occur. The sugar will help prevent the production of ketones. Therefore, you should substitute your usual carbohydrate intake with drinks, such as Lucozade or sweetened fruit juices. Take a glassful at hourly intervals. A list of suitable fluid foods to take when ill is given below.

Alternatives to solid food

Lucozade, fruit juice, fizzy drinks, milk, soup, ice cream, Complan, drinking chocolate, sugar/glucose, honey/jam/syrup

---

STEP 2 – take some tests

When you start feeling ill you must do tests to see whether your blood glucose is rising. Blood tests are clearly more helpful than urine in this respect and give you an accurate picture, although it may be useful to check the urine for the presence of ketones. You should test at least four times a day until you feel better. If you are changing the insulin dose, more frequent tests may be helpful, say every two hours. Unfortunately, when you are ill you will probably not feel like doing these tests. However, during an illness the results of your tests are particularly important. Remember, your blood glucose may be rising and your dose of insulin may need adjusting.

STEP 3 – adjust your insulin dose

- NEVER STOP TAKING YOUR INSULIN, however ill you feel, or however little you are eating. Remember, even if you stop eating and continue to take your usual dose of insulin, it is very unlikely that you will become hypoglycaemic when you are ill. The body will automatically provide glucose from its stores and it is more likely that the glucose will rise.
- If the blood glucose is less than 10 mmol/l, continue with your usual insulin dose.
- If the blood glucose is greater than 12 mmol/l, then your insulin dose should be increased. As a general rule, an increase less than a quarter of your normal dose is usually ineffective. If your normal dose is less than 8 units per dose, a 2 unit increase is usually sufficient. A 4 to 8 unit increase would be suitable for somebody taking 20 to 30 units per dose. For those on 40 units a 10 unit increase would be better.

STEP 4 – check again

■ If after about four hours you are still feeling unwell, you should check your blood glucose again. If it is higher than 12 mmol/l (or your urine is still full of glucose) you can take some more quick-acting insulin, say another 4 to 8 units. Again use quick-acting insulin.

■ It is probably sensible to continue on quick-acting insulin alone, repeated every four to six hours, until you are feeling better.

■ If you normally only use slow-acting insulin or mixtures, the same principles can apply. If the blood glucose is normal, continue your normal dose. If it is high, increase the dose. However, if the illness continues for more than a few hours a switch to quick-acting insulin will be necessary. It is wise to be prepared for this. Ask your doctor to give you some quick-acting insulin to use if necessary.

■ If after a few hours you are still vomiting, or have become very thirsty, and your tests are high you MUST obtain expert advice and should seek medical help, especially if ketones are present in your urine.

■ If you have had problems with dealing with illness, it might be worth asking your doctor or specialist nurse about testing for ketones. This may help you from getting into difficulties again.

Summary

These steps may seem rather complicated. The first time that an illness of this kind occurs it is probably sensible to talk it through with your specialist nurse or doctor. Certainly you should discuss the possibility with them and establish exactly the types of insulin you should take and the sorts of dose increases that would suit you best. Partners or friends may worry too, so include them in your discussions.

■ Hypoglycaemia

When the balance is wrong

Good diabetes control depends on establishing and maintaining a balance between the meals you eat and your injections of insulin. On occasions you may get this balance wrong (see graphs above). This might occur, for example, when you have an unusually small meal, you omit your between meal snacks or you take unexpected exercise. There may be too much insulin

GOOD DIABETIC CONTROL IS A MATTER OF BALANCE

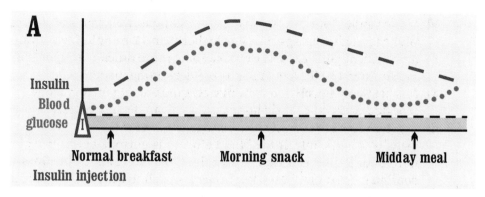

Regular meals and regular insulin injections lead to the ideal balance
between insulin and blood glucose

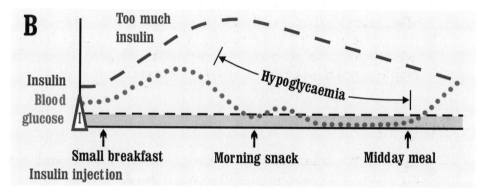

Poor balance can occur after an unusually small meal

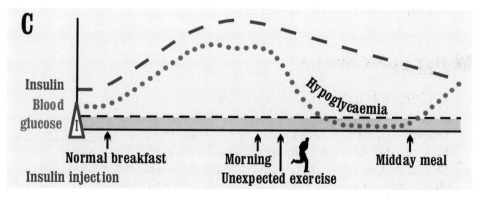

Unexpected exercise rapidly lowers the blood glucose, causing an imbalance

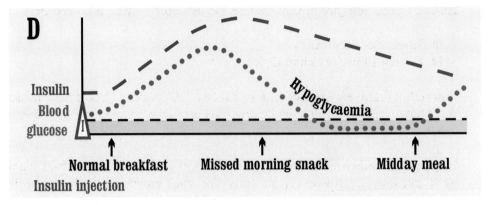

D

Insulin
Blood
glucose

Hypoglycaemia

Normal breakfast   Missed morning snack   Midday meal
Insulin injection

Missing a between meals snack causes a reduced blood glucose level

in proportion to the amount of glucose in the blood. As a result your blood glucose will fall too low. This is called hypoglycaemia, a hypo, a hypoglycaemic or insulin reaction (or just a reaction). Normally you develop symptoms that you will easily recognise.

You can take simple steps that will put these conditions right. If you do not respond to these symptoms they may progress to unconsciousness. Therefore, it is important that you are able to:

■ Recognise when hypoglycaemia is occurring
■ Take steps to put it right
■ Prevent it from happening again.

■ Recognising hypoglycaemia

The common symptoms of hypoglycaemia include:

■ Trembling
■ Sweating
■ Tingling around the mouth
■ Palpitations of the heart
■ Difficulty in concentration
■ Confusion
■ Muzziness

■ Faintness
■ Headache
■ Blurring of vision
■ Unsteadiness
■ Irritability, bad temper
■ Unusual lack of co-operation
■ Vomiting (occasionally in children).

If the correct steps are not taken, these symptoms may be followed by:

- Loss of consciousness
- Convulsions (occasionally).

You will usually experience one or more of the early symptoms. It is likely that these same symptoms will occur each time your blood glucose becomes too low.

If hypoglycaemia occurs at night, the early symptoms will normally wake you up. Occasionally, however, the only sign that your glucose has been low during the night may be a headache on waking in the morning.

But what happens if you fail to notice the initial symptoms (for example, during the night), and you therefore go into a hypoglycaemic coma? Fortunately, your body will eventually recognise what has happened, and will start to make sufficient glucose to bring about recovery. Death or disability does not often occur as a result of hypoglycaemia, except when very large overdoses of insulin are given or large amounts of alcohol have been consumed.

■ Treatment of hypoglycaemia

Immediate treatment will rapidly restore you to normal. It is important that AS SOON AS THE WARNING SYMPTOMS OCCUR, you:

- STOP what you are doing. This is especially important when driving or using moving machinery.
- IMMEDIATELY take two lumps of sugar, three glucose tablets, two teaspoonfuls of sugar in squash together with a couple of biscuits (the amount needed is usually 10–20 grams). Within a few minutes the symptoms should have disappeared, but if not, take another two glucose tablets.

Three essential precautions

1. ALWAYS carry some form of sugar which can be swallowed easily as soon as you experience any symptoms of hypoglycaemia.

2. ALWAYS carry some identification to say that you have diabetes treated with insulin. If you should fail to experience the warning symptoms and become unconscious, it is essential that anybody who discovers you should recognise that you have diabetes. Therefore, carry a card, such as the Identity Card produced by Diabetes UK, which provides clear instructions about the action that should be taken.

3. ALWAYS inform those who might need to know, such as workmates, relatives, teachers, etc, that there is a possibility that you could become hypoglycaemic. Try not to feel embarrassed about this. If they can recognise the early symptoms, it may save the possibly more embarrassing situation where you pass out unexpectedly!

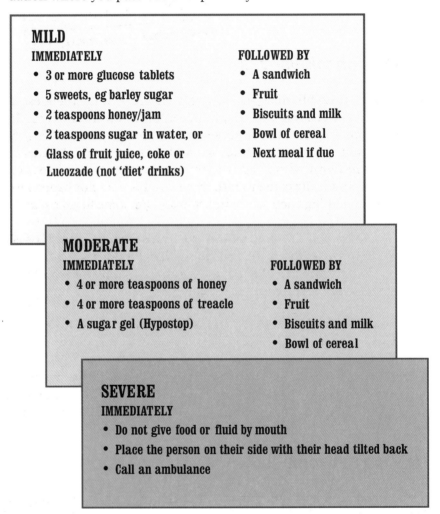

MILD
IMMEDIATELY
- 3 or more glucose tablets
- 5 sweets, eg barley sugar
- 2 teaspoons honey/jam
- 2 teaspoons sugar in water, or
- Glass of fruit juice, coke or Lucozade (not 'diet' drinks)

FOLLOWED BY
- A sandwich
- Fruit
- Biscuits and milk
- Bowl of cereal
- Next meal if due

MODERATE
IMMEDIATELY
- 4 or more teaspoons of honey
- 4 or more teaspoons of treacle
- A sugar gel (Hypostop)

FOLLOWED BY
- A sandwich
- Fruit
- Biscuits and milk
- Bowl of cereal

SEVERE
IMMEDIATELY
- Do not give food or fluid by mouth
- Place the person on their side with their head tilted back
- Call an ambulance

Foods and fluids which may be used to treat hypoglycaemia

Always carry some form
of identification

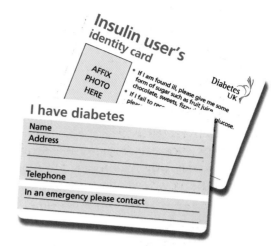

Losing consciousness

Sometimes, possibly unavoidably, you may lose consciousness due to a hypoglycaemic reaction. You will, however, always recover. When the blood glucose drops this low the body responds by making glucose. This, however, may not occur quickly enough to stop you passing out. With time, however, the natural response of the body will restore the blood glucose to normal and you will automatically come round. Provided this does not happen when you are doing something such as driving, you should come to no harm.

Occasionally, when this occurs, you may have a convulsion. This is a quite natural response by the body. It does not indicate that you have developed epilepsy. Remember that there are steps that other people can take to help bring you round more quickly (see below).

Brain damage and death are almost unheard of in those experiencing occasional loss of consciousness.

More care is needed with children under the age of five, when frequent severe reactions may be harmful. Very elderly people, living on their own, should also be more careful, as they are more likely to come to harm if they pass out.

What other people should do

Companions can help you to come round more quickly. If you are actually unconscious, people should NOT try to give you sugar drinks as you may not be able to swallow these.

They may try Hypostop. This is a jelly-like material containing sugar, which can be smeared on the gums under the lips (not in the mouth between the teeth). Some of the sugar will be absorbed, and will help bring your blood glucose up more quickly. However, it should not be used if you are unconscious and unable to swallow.

Glucagon injection

There is an injection called glucagon. This has the opposite effect to insulin. It causes the blood glucose to rise and consciousness is rapidly regained. The injection is very easy to give. It does not have to be given by a doctor. Friends, colleagues or family members can easily learn the technique. It does not matter whether the needle penetrates the blood vessel. It just works more quickly and does no harm. It is in fact best delivered into a muscle area. The needle therefore is a little longer than that used for insulin injection.

A special kit is provided for glucagon. You can obtain this on prescription but your companions should be shown how to use the kit by a diabetes specialist nurse or a doctor. Sometimes people feel a little sick or actually vomit after the injection but these feelings soon pass.

What you should do when you recover

As soon as you come round from a hypo, you must have something to eat. This is especially important if somebody has helped you, since the sugar or glucagon that they have given may only have a short-term effect. But even with less severe hypos there may still be too much insulin around. This could cause you to have another hypo later. If you have a sandwich, two or three digestive biscuits, or something else containing longer-acting carbohydrate, this will ensure that you are all right. Test your blood glucose regularly for the rest of the day. Sometimes the effect of the injection may be prolonged and you will need a further top-up of carbohydrate.

If you have had a bad reaction, your warning senses may be temporarily blunted for a day or so. We would suggest, therefore, that you reduce your insulin dosages for 48 hours after a bad reaction. This will allow your blood glucose to run a little on the high side. This will ensure that your warning symptoms are restored.

There may be a rebound of your blood glucose after a bad reaction. This means that your glucose levels will remain automatically a bit high for several hours, or possibly a day or so after such a reaction. Do not try to correct this immediately by increasing your insulin again. Just give yourself a day or so of space. Running slightly high for a day or so will do you no harm. After two or three days you can get back to normal.

Advice to give your companions

It is important that your relatives, friends and work colleagues should recognise when you are suffering from hypoglycaemia, particularly if you are unaware of it and not taking the right steps. They should be instructed to take the following action:

■ Stop you from continuing with any potentially dangerous activity.

■ Persuade you to take some glucose tablets, sugar, or a sweet drink, such as Lucozade or Ribena (NOT low-calorie drinks) followed by something more substantial like a sandwich, fruit, biscuits and milk or a bowl of cereal.

■ If this is unsuccessful and you become incoherent or confused, they should try putting a spoonful of honey, treacle or a glucose gel (Hypostop) into the side of your mouth and rubbing it into your cheek. This needs to be followed up as you recover by something more substantial as above.

■ If you should become unconscious, they MUST NOT try to give you sugar by mouth, but should call a doctor or ambulance and put you on your side with head tilted back.

■ Alternatively, they may be taught to give glucagon, but this is only necessary if you are subject to unexpected attacks of hypoglycaemia which cause unconsciousness (details described above). As soon as you regain consciousness, they should make sure you take something sugary followed by something more substantial as above, because the effect of glucagon is only temporary.

■ Try not to be embarrassed about telling other people about your diabetes. It may be much more difficult if no one recognises when you are going low and you then pass out!

■ Preventing hypoglycaemia

You will almost inevitably experience some mild hypos if you are achieving good control. These should be easily recognised.

However, you will want to avoid bad hypoglycaemic reactions. Not only are they unpleasant and embarrassing, but also they could be dangerous if, for example, you are driving, or operating machinery.

Remember, hypoglycaemic reactions will occur when there is no longer a balance between your blood glucose and the insulin you inject. The commonest times are:

- Mid-morning or before lunch
- During the night
- After exercise.

Night hypoglycaemia

Night hypoglycaemia usually occurs when using a mixture of quick- and slow-acting insulin, either together before your evening meal or the quick before your evening meal and the slow at bedtime.

Reduction of slow-acting insulin may eliminate the hypos but result in a high blood sugar in the morning.

The reason for night hypoglycaemic reactions is that there is an overlap between quick-acting insulin, which may last 5–7 hours, and slow-acting insulins. This results in too much insulin in the blood at 2–3 am, causing hypoglycaemia.

With very quick-acting insulins which only last 2–4 hours the effects have worn off by bedtime. There is no overlap, therefore no reaction. If morning blood sugars remain high it is then safe to increase the slow-acting insulin to deal with this.

Exercise and hypoglycaemia

How can exercise cause hypoglycaemia?

When you take exercise, your muscles use up glucose at a more rapid rate than when your muscles are at rest. If you have taken your normal insulin dose and eaten the usual amount, a hypoglycaemic reaction can occur (see graph C on page 113). This can be prevented, however, by following one of two courses of action:

■ Take extra carbohydrate and/or

■ Reduce your insulin dosage beforehand.

Taking extra carbohydrate

If you take any form of exercise, you will quickly learn how much extra carbo-hydrate you will need. This amount is very individual and will depend on the duration and intensity of exercise, how fit you are and when you last ate. As a general guideline, it is recommended that you increase your carbohydrate intake gradually and monitor the effect. If the activity is prolonged or very strenuous, a further additional carbohydrate may be required, eg sugary drinks, chocolate such as a Mars bar, bread or biscuits. You will also need to take extra carbohydrate, eg potato, bread or pasta, at the meal after you have exercised.

The effect of exercise may be delayed. This explains why sometimes, even though extra carbohydrate may have been taken before, during and after exercise, you may experience a hypoglycaemic reaction several hours later (or even the following morning). This is particularly likely to happen with strenuous exercise, such as regular training for sports. If, therefore, you have taken such exercise, for example in the early evening, you should always check a test two to three hours later, say before you go to bed, in case you need an extra top-up of carbohydrate.

Performing regular blood tests will help you to work out the times when you are most likely to be hypoglycaemic. This will allow you to take preventive action.

Reducing your insulin dosage

Reducing your insulin dose may be preferable when you know that extra exercise or strenuous work is expected. You need to learn, therefore, to think ahead a bit. For example, regular daily work, Monday to Friday, especially that involving steady physical exercise (eg bricklaying or gardening), can be best coped with by reducing the morning insulin on working days. You can then increase the dose when you might be less active, for example at weekends. The same principle applies, for example, for regular sporting activities, eg physical education periods at school. In the case of very strenuous activities, this will need to be combined with extra carbohydrate.

In contrast, the sedentary worker might take normal doses of insulin during the week, but for active gardeners the dose of insulin might be reduced at the weekend.

For children, an adjustment of insulin dosage may be necessary at weekends, or when they return to school after the holidays.

If you are using multiple injections (pen regimen) for controlling your insulin, you will certainly learn to anticipate what you are likely to be doing in the few hours after each injection. The aim will be to reduce the insulin, for example, at lunch-time, if you know that you are going to have a busy afternoon, or if you are going to have less to eat at that meal than usual.

Loss of warning symptoms

This is probably the most frightening experience that may occur. This of course is when you become unconscious without feeling any of the warning symptoms and without being able to take action to prevent it. There are three circumstances under which this may occur.

1. If you have had one bad reaction then, for the next day or so, the warning symptoms may be blunted. Therefore, after such a reaction, it is a good idea to allow yourself, by reducing your insulin dose slightly, to run your blood glucose a little higher than usual, say around 11 mmol/l, for a day or two to get back to normal. Discuss this with your diabetes care team.
2. After many years of diabetes the body may become resistant to the warning signs. This usually only occurs after fifteen or twenty years of diabetes. It certainly does not occur in everybody. Indeed, four out of five people never experience this.

    Lack of awareness may occur because you have been a little over-strict with your glucose control and running consistently too low. If you should reach the stage where you feel that you are becoming very low without getting any warning signs, then you will have to be careful to take more frequent tests. This usually enables you to avoid any serious problems.
3. It can also occur if you take strenuous exercise using the muscles in the area that you have recently injected, or, rarely, because you inadvertently inject into a blood vessel.

◼ General approach and attitudes

Do remember that even bad reactions rarely cause you harm. They can, of course, cause you some embarrassment, but this is likely to be less if those close to you know about the problem and its causes. This is one good reason for being open with your family, friends and work colleagues about your diabetes. The more they, and even employers, know about your diabetes, the less likely they are to react badly or inappropriately. Do try not to be too defensive about reactions.

If you over-react all the time by running your blood glucose too high continuously (not just for a day or two), then you do run the risk, after several years, of the much more serious complications of diabetes. These are those that involve your eyes, kidneys and feet.

Some final comments

To prevent reactions, the aim must be to maintain the balance. Therefore, make sure that you:

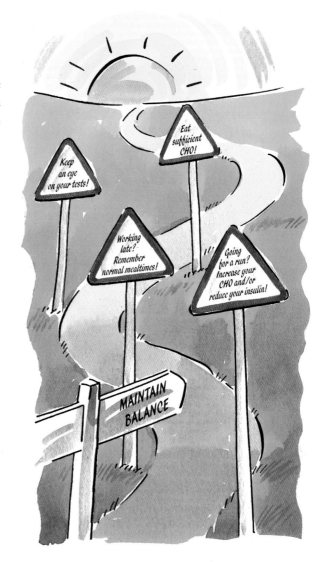

If, having checked that none of the above apply, you still have frequent reactions, an increase in your food, or a reduction in insulin dose, may be necessary.

Remember:

- ■ Very quick-acting insulin reaches its maximum one to two hours after injection.
- ■ Quick-acting insulin reaches its maximum four to six hours after an injection, ie midday after a 7.30 am injection, or midnight after an evening injection.
- ■ Slow-acting insulin reaches its maximum six to ten hours after an injection, ie mid-afternoon, or in the early hours of the morning.

■ A word of warning

Although the aim is to prevent hypoglycaemia, you must not achieve this by running a constantly high blood glucose. A high blood glucose may ensure against hypoglycaemic reactions, but over a prolonged period it will cause serious and permanent damage.

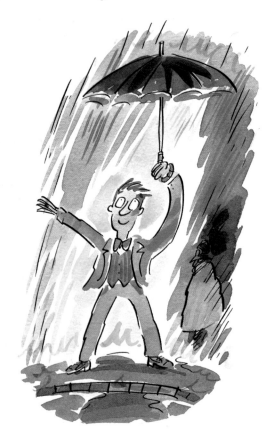

8 The Long-Term Effects of Diabetes and Your General Health

This chapter describes the possible long-term effects of diabetes, how they may affect you, and the sort of treatment that can be given. An outline is also provided of the type of medical care and supervision you should expect.

Treatment of diabetes very rapidly restores health to normal. The symptoms disappear quite quickly and any loss of weight or energy soon returns to normal.

After many years of diabetes, however, some of the body's tissues may be damaged. The eyes, kidneys and some nerves (mainly those to the feet) are most susceptible. In addition, there is an increased risk of damage to the circulation, potentially leading to heart disease and stroke. Care with other aspects of your health, regular attendance for monitoring and, if necessary, treatment should keep these risks to a minimum. These problems are likely to develop only after many years of poor blood glucose control. Therefore, they are preventable by the majority of people. Many are completely spared these problems and, even after more than 40 years of diabetes, show no trace of any complications.

■ Damage to the eyes

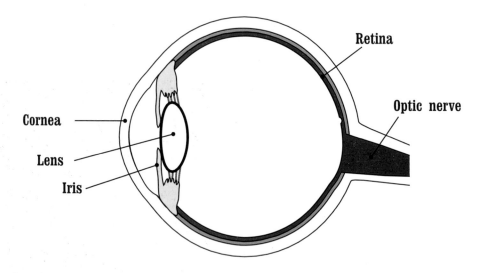

The parts of the eye

Two parts of the eye are affected by diabetes.

1. The lens: Opacities in the lens (cataracts) are common in elderly people and sometimes cause deterioration of vision. Cataracts are more common in older people with diabetes.
2. The retina: This is the sensitive part of the back of the eye. The damage that can be caused by diabetes is called diabetic retinopathy. This takes several years to develop. It is extremely rare in children. Usually abnormalities are minor and cause no loss of vision. In a minority of sufferers, however, this retinopathy can progress and vision can deteriorate. Without early treatment the affected eye may become blind, usually from bleeding (haemorrhage) within the eye.

Prevention and treatment of eye damage

Cataracts can interfere with vision. However, in the early stages they may cause no problems. They will, if present, be detected at your routine yearly eye examination. If this is the case do not be too alarmed. It may be several years before they interfere with vision. When this happens they can be treated by a simple and straightforward operation. A new artificial lens will almost always restore sight to normal.

Damage to the retina can fortunately now be treated. Blindness should not occur. Treatment is by laser, a process which involves aiming a fine beam of very bright light at the abnormal blood vessel. It is simple to perform and is usually successful. But it does have to be undertaken before sight has deteriorated too seriously. Therefore, it is essential that you have your pupils dilated and the back of your eyes examined regularly – ideally annually. This can be done by an optician, by doctors in the diabetic clinic or by an eye specialist.

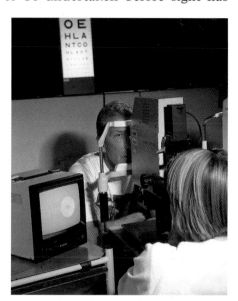

Finally, some blurring of vision may occur in the first few weeks of treatment for diabetes. This is usually of no consequence and nearly always resolves within a week or two, so do not get your glasses changed. Subsequently, if you should notice a sudden loss of vision in either eye, you must report it to your doctor immediately.

Contact lenses

People with diabetes should be aware that they have a higher risk of developing irritation of the eye from contact lens use than those without diabetes. A meticulous cleaning routine and careful technique for lens handling are important. You should make sure you have been shown how to do this and you should have your technique checked from time to time. If you are using daily-wear soft lenses, these should be exchanged every six months.

Extended-wear soft lenses should not be generally prescribed for those with diabetes, as damage to the cornea is more common with this type. If your eyes become red or irritated, you should immediately stop using contact lenses and seek advice.

■ Damage to the feet

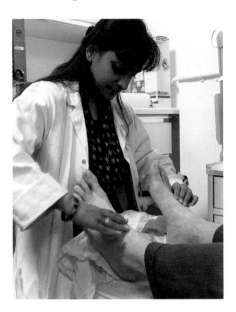

After a number of years of diabetes the feet can be damaged in two ways:

1. Damage to the nerves (called neuropathy or neuritis) may occur. This mainly affects the sensation in the feet. The problem is that those in whom it occurs may not be aware of the subtle loss of feeling in their feet. The feet normally undergo a lot of wear and tear and any injuries are usually noticed because they hurt. However, injuries may not be painful because of neuropathy, and increasing damage may pass unnoticed. Ulceration and infection can be very serious. They can result in prolonged periods off work and sometimes require operations, or even amputations. However, these injuries can, to a large extent, be avoided if proper care is taken of the feet.

2. Damage to the blood vessels to the feet. As people become middle-aged or elderly, there tends to be some deterioration in the blood vessels of the body, including those in the legs and feet. This is slightly more likely if you have diabetes – especially if you smoke! This, also, will be looked for at your yearly examination by the doctor, who will warn you if a problem is detected. In serious cases symptoms develop. These are: cramping pains in the calves or thighs on walking which are relieved when you stop, and severe persistent pain which comes on suddenly in the feet or lower leg. If this happens, and especially if the feet are discoloured, you should report immediately to your doctor. Fortunately these problems can usually be relieved by a variety of procedures to restore the circulation.

Prevention of foot problems

For young people

In young people, ie those under 30 and especially those who have had diabetes for fewer than 15 years, neuropathy and circulation problems are very unlikely. They are virtually unknown in children. Therefore simple and general care of the feet (as for any other young people) is all that is required.

This includes:

■ Choosing shoes which are comfortable and fit well.
■ Keeping the feet clean.
■ Taking medical advice if you develop ingrowing toenails, infection of the feet and, especially, any ulceration.

For older people and those with early nerve damage or circulatory problems

As you get older, and the longer you have diabetes, the chances of developing neuropathy and circulation problems increase a bit. You should be checked yearly for these and your doctor should tell you if there are any signs of this sort of damage. If so, follow the steps described below.

For those with definite neuropathy or circulatory problems and the elderly

These recommendations are essential. You should read them carefully. Scrupulous care can prevent serious problems.

Inspecting your feet

■ Inspect your feet regularly – ideally, daily – and if you cannot do this yourself, ask a friend to do it for you. If you are doing this on your own, a mirror on the floor or by the skirting board may help you to see. This inspection is important because you may not always be able to feel bruises or sores.

■ Seek advice if you develop any cracks or breaks in the skin, any calluses or corns, or your feet are swollen or throbbing. Advice from a state registered chiropodist is freely available under the NHS.

Washing your feet

■ Wash your feet daily in warm water. There is no advantage in soaking your feet – this makes the skin soggy at first and then dry, and more likely to become damaged.

■ Use a mild type of soap

■ Rinse the skin well after washing. Dry your feet carefully, blotting between the toes with a soft towel.

■ Dust with plain talc and wipe off any excess, so that it does not clog between the toes

■ Use moisturising cream after bathing, but do not apply cream between your toes as this area is usually moist enough.

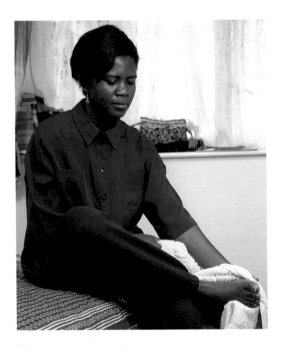

Nail cutting

■ When the toenails need cutting, do this after bathing, when the nails are soft and pliable. Do not cut them too short.

■ Never cut the corners of your nails too far back at the sides, but allow the cut to follow the natural line of the end of the toe.

■ Never use a sharp instrument to clean under your nails or in the nail grooves at the sides of the nails.

■ If your toenails are painful, or if you experience difficulty in cutting them, consult your chiropodist.

Heat and cold

- Be careful to avoid baths that are too hot.
- Do not sit too close to heaters or fires.
- Before getting into bed, remove hot water bottles, unless they are fabric covered. Electric underblankets should be switched off or unplugged.
- If your feet get wet, dry them, and put on dry socks as soon as possible.
- Do not use hot fomentations or poultices.

Shoes

Shoes must fit properly and provide adequate support. In fact, careful fitting and choice of shoes is probably the most important measure you can take to prevent diabetic foot problems. Therefore:

- Wear well fitting shoes. They must be comfortable.
- Never accept shoes that have to be 'broken-in' before becoming comfortable.
- When buying new shoes, always try them on, and rely on the advice of a qualified shoe fitter. Shoes must always be the correct shape for your feet.
- Slippers do not provide adequate support and therefore should be worn only for short periods (night and morning), and not throughout the day.
- Do not wear garters.
- Avoid walking barefoot.
- Daily rule – Feel inside your shoes and slippers before putting them on. This is important because you may not feel nails or stones under your feet as a result of loss of sensitivity in your feet.

Corns and calluses

- Do not cut corns and calluses yourself, or let a well meaning friend cut them for you, seek help of a state registered chiropodist.
- Do not use corn paints or corn plasters. They contain caustic materials which can be extremely damaging to those with diabetes.

First aid measures

- Minor injuries, such as cuts and abrasions, can be self-treated quite adequately, by gently cleaning the area with soap and water and covering them with a sterile dressing.
- If blisters occur, do not prick them. If they burst, dress them as for a minor cut.
- Never use strong medicaments, such as iodine, Dettol, Germolene or other powerful antiseptics.
- Never place adhesive strapping directly over a wound.
- If you are in the slightest doubt about how to deal with any wound, discoloration, corns, and especially ulcers, consult your doctor.

■ Painful neuropathy

Sometimes diabetic neuropathy causes pain. This is usually in the feet and legs and is particularly disagreeable. It builds up gradually. Typically, it causes a burning sensation, a feeling of pins and needles, with unpleasant discomfort on contact with clothes or bedclothes. It is usually worse in bed at night. Unpleasant though most of these symptoms are, they almost always disappear in time. However, it can, unfortunately, take many months for them to do so. Very good diabetic control is essential. Various treatments will help relieve the pain. Specialist advice is recommended.

■ Sexual function

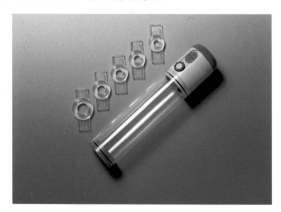

Nerve damage can cause difficulty with erections (impotence). However, impotence is also common in those without diabetes. It is said that as many as 50 per cent of middle-aged men have quite long (but often temporary) periods of difficulty with erection. It is often due to psychological factors. For this reason, if you do have this problem, it may be difficult to be absolutely sure whether or not it is due to the nerve damage resulting from diabetes. Proper diagnosis is important and specialist advice should be sought from your doctor or from trained counsellors.

A variety of treatments are now available and these can be very successful. They include Viagra, injections and treatments which can be given into the penis or a variety of devices which may produce an erection. In severe cases there are some operations which can help.

Although it may seem embarrassing, do not hesitate to tell your doctor if you are concerned about this problem. Only in this way can a proper diagnosis be reached, with referral to an expert who should be able to help.

■ Other rare problems due to neuropathy

Occasionally the part of the nervous system which controls the bowel, bladder and some other functions of the body may be damaged by diabetes.

With regard to the bowel, a rather unusual type of diarrhoea may develop. This tends to be explosive and particularly occurs at night. Fortunately it is usually quite intermittent.

Occasionally the nerves to the stomach may be affected. This causes delay of emptying and may cause nausea and sometimes vomiting.

The bladder may likewise be affected, giving rise to some difficulty in emptying the bladder when passing urine.

Finally, the control of the blood pressure may be partially affected. This is usually manifested by a slight dizziness when you stand up.

It should be stressed that these are very unusual complications and they only occur after many years of diabetes. Special treatments are now available which help to relieve these problems. Therefore if you feel you have symptoms which concern you, do tell your doctor about them.

■ Damage to the kidneys

Damage to the kidneys (usually called nephropathy) occurs less frequently than eye damage. The injuries to the kidneys must have been present for many years before function begins to deteriorate. Even then a few more years usually elapse before the situation becomes serious. Unfortunately kidney disease does not give rise to symptoms until it is quite advanced. Early detection by means of regular checks from your doctor is very important. There is a test that can be performed on your urine which gives an indication of early damage. These tests become positive at a stage when the situation can usually still be put right.

■ Arterial disease and high blood pressure

Degeneration or hardening and narrowing of the arteries (blood vessels) are normal consequences of ageing. With diabetes, however, there may be some acceleration of this process. This may cause poor circulation in the feet and legs and can contribute to heart attack or stroke.

High blood pressure

High blood pressure (hypertension) is more common in people with diabetes. We now recognise that it is particularly important for this to be treated, especially in those with diabetes. This will reduce the risk of heart attack or stroke. Indeed, the standards set for treatment of blood pressure for those with diabetes are now rather more strict than for those without.

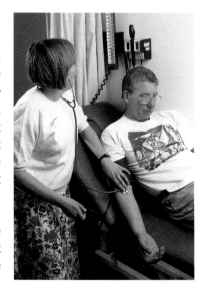

There is a wide range of tablets which can be used and it is uncommon to fail to find a tablet or combination of tablets which can treat the blood pressure without significant side-effects. Several of these tablets have a specific effect in preventing damage to your blood vessels from the effects of normal wear and tear and the diabetes itself.

Side-effects of tablets, if they do occur, depend on the type of tablet. One commonly used tablet sometimes causes an irritating cough. This is relieved when the tablet is changed. Another may produce slightly cold hands and feet and should be avoided in those with asthma. Details of side-effects should always be included on the information leaflet provided by your pharmacist. For legal reasons all possible side-effects are listed, however rare. But most people suffer no side-effects at all. If in doubt discuss this with your doctor before starting treatment.

Blood pressure does go up and down during the day. To achieve maximum benefit you need 24-hour control. Therefore, you should try to take the tablets at the times recommended.

Weight control and regular, and hopefully pleasurable, exercise help keep your blood pressure down. Smoking, however, has the reverse effect.

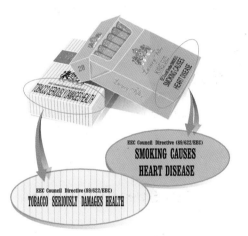

We recommend, therefore, that:

- Your blood pressure is checked at least annually
- You keep as good control of your weight as possible
- You avoid or stop smoking
- You try to take regular exercise
- If tablets are prescribed, you take them in the dose and at the time recommended.

The steps that you can take yourself may not only prevent the blood pressure rising but also, if it does need treating, help limit the number of tablets needed to keep it in the normal range. Side-effects of any tablets are therefore much less likely.

Blood cholesterol

A raised cholesterol level in the blood may aggravate a tendency to develop arterial disease. If the diabetes is poorly controlled the blood cholesterol is raised. In some individuals it is high, even when the blood glucose is normal. Over the age of 40 you should ask for a test (every five years). If it is persistently high, tablets are available which should help bring the level down to normal.

■ Diabetes and other illnesses

The effect of illness on diabetes

In the section on treatment (Chapter 3) it was indicated that under certain circumstances your diabetes may go temporarily out of control. Although loss of control for a few days is of no real significance, if you should develop symptoms of thirst and dryness of the mouth, or pass large quantities of urine, you should consult your doctor.

Remember:

1. If you develop nausea or vomiting you must follow the rules on page 110.
2. Since any illness usually causes your blood glucose to rise, do increase your insulin. Never reduce or stop it.

Diabetes and the treatment of other illnesses

Diabetes is no bar to the treatment – including operations – of any other disorder or illness. Your diabetes may not be so easily controlled during any illness or after an operation. Adjustment of your diabetes treatment may be necessary.

Dentistry

Straightforward, routine dental treatment can be carried out by your dentist in the normal way. When the treatment involves general anaesthesia, however, this should always be performed by a hospital team and not in the dental surgery.

For all dental procedures, INSULIN MUST BE ADMINISTERED AS USUAL – it must not be stopped or reduced for fear that insufficient food will be taken to balance it. The reason for this is that the stress of the procedure is likely to raise the blood glucose, rather than lower it.

Sometimes after dental treatment you may be unable to eat normally. You should take fluids containing sugar in equivalent amounts to your normal needs, until you are eating normally again. Should you have any doubts about a planned dental procedure, discuss it with your doctor before going ahead.

Diabetic control whilst in hospital

When you are in hospital you are often confined to bed and will be taking less exercise than usual. You will probably be anxious, and your diet may be different. Together, these factors will undoubtedly cause your blood glucose to rise. Consequently, your insulin dose will need to be increased. You should realise that these changes are the result of prevailing circumstances. It is not a failure on your part or on the part of the hospital staff.

Unless you are very unwell you may prefer to continue to look after your diabetes yourself. This is perfectly permissible. Ask the nursing staff if you can do this. Also remind them and the doctors that you would like any changes in your diabetes treatment to be explained and discussed with you.

If you are not able to eat and drink normally your diabetes can be very easily controlled. This is done by giving insulin and glucose through a vein via an intravenous drip. This is quite routine and easy to do. It ensures that your diabetes will cause you no problems until you are better.

If you are admitted to hospital for any reason, you should make sure that your diabetes care team is informed.

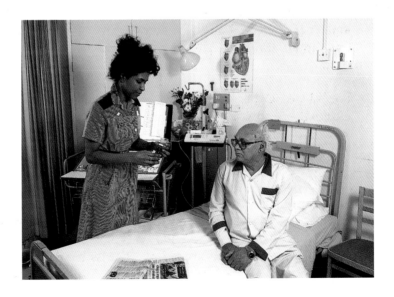

■ Clinic attendance

The organisation of clinics

Your local diabetes clinic plays an important role in the treatment and control of your diabetes. The organisation of these clinics varies in different areas of the country. In the majority of cases the clinic is at the local hospital and is under the direction of a hospital consultant. Many units have set up special diabetes centres with expertly trained doctors, nurses, dietitians and chiropodists. In many districts clinics have been established in specially trained general practices, or cooperative schemes have been developed between hospital specialists and family doctors. Evening clinics may be held to enable you to attend after work.

■ Regular medical review

In the period after your diabetes has been diagnosed, your doctor may wish to see you every few weeks, until he or she is sure that the treatment is effective. However, when your blood glucose has been brought under control, you may only need to attend perhaps every few months.

With your blood (or urine) test records you will be able to keep a routine check on the effectiveness of your treatment. None the less, from time to time it is essential that you visit your doctor or clinic so that your treatment can be monitored, and any specific problems you may have can be dealt with.

- Your doctor will want to be sure that your tests are satisfactory. If the record of your tests shows erratic or high glucose levels, he or she will decide whether additional treatment is necessary.
- You should have the long-term averaging test (HbA_{1c} or fructos-amine). This gives an indication of your overall average blood glucose control (see page 75).
- Your doctor will want to ensure that you understand and are happy with the advice you have been given. This is the time for you to ask questions!
- From time to time, you do have to be checked to see whether any long-term complications have developed. It is important that these should be detected before you notice anything wrong, so that early treatment can be commenced.

■ Finally, such visits provide you with an opportunity to discuss problems with, for example, your dietitian. You should also report any new symptoms, such as difficulty with vision or problems with your feet.

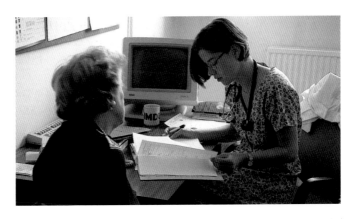

Once your diabetes is reasonably controlled you should:

1. See a specialist nurse, doctor, dietitian and chiropodist at regular intervals – annually, or more often if necessary. These meetings should give time for discussion as well as for assessing your control.
2. Be able to contact any member of the healthcare team for specialist advice when you need it.
3. Have more education sessions as you are ready for them.
4. Have a formal medical review at least once a year by a doctor experienced in diabetes. This review should include the following.

■ Your weight should be recorded.
■ Your urine should be tested for protein.
■ Your blood should be tested to measure long-term control.
■ You should discuss control, including your home monitoring results.
■ Your blood pressure should be checked.
■ Your vision should be checked, and the backs of your eyes examined. To do this your pupils have to be dilated. This requires some drops to be put into your eyes. This is in no way harmful. They may sting a bit for a minute or so. However, you need to be warned that there may be some blurring of vision for a while after this. You are advised, therefore, not to drive on this occasion, or if you do you must be careful. It can be particularly uncomfortable if it is a very bright day, and you would be advised to use some dark glasses. The blurring wears off, usually within quite a short time, and no long-term effects occur.

- Your legs and feet should be examined to check your circulation and nerve supply. If necessary you should be referred to a chiropodist.
- Your injection sites should be examined.
- You should have the opportunity to discuss how you are coping at home and at work.
- Beyond the age of 40 it is wise to have your cholesterol checked. If the result is normal, this test only needs to be repeated every five years.

The control of your diabetes is important, and so are the detection and treatment of any complications. Make sure you are getting the medical care and education you need to ensure you stay healthy. If you are not feeling well, your treatment appears not to be working, or you develop any unusual symptoms such as worsening eyesight, or abnormal tingling in the hands or feet, report them to your doctor at once – DO NOT WAIT FOR YOUR NEXT APPOINTMENT.

OUTPATIENT APPOINTMENTS

Name _____

Address _____

_____

Date	Time	Consultant	Clinic

Bring this card with you to the hospital

■ Summary

It must be stressed that the problems of long-term diabetes occur only in a minority of people with diabetes.

Remember:

- ■ Good control of diabetes usually prevents the development of these complications. Therefore, advice from regular clinic attendance is very important.
- ■ Smoking accelerates arterial disease (affecting the heart and feet), and may also have a bad effect on your eyes and kidneys.
- ■ Try to control your weight.
- ■ Keep a regular eye on your own tests.

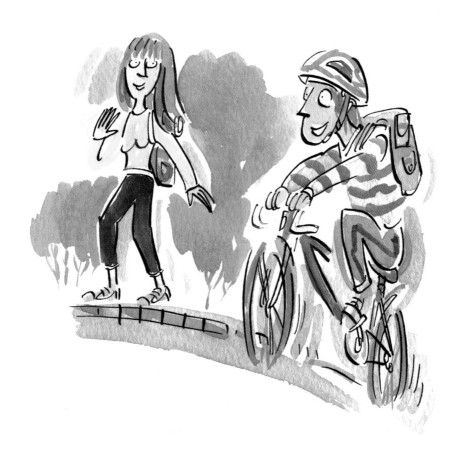

9 Sexual Relationships Pregnancy, Parenthood and Contraception

Sex, marriage and parenthood are likely to be part of normal life. This chapter answers some of the questions you might have on these topics.

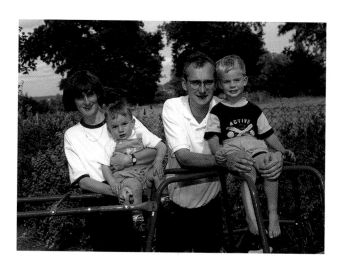

Diabetes should not prevent you from forming a relationship and having a family

■ Sexual development and relationships

You may often worry about the possibility that your diabetes may prevent you from having a normal sexual life. However, worry is far more likely to upset your sex life than the diabetes! If your diabetes is well controlled, you should have no more problems than anybody else.

Puberty will occur normally – almost everybody feels that they have not developed as well as others of the same age, whether they have diabetes or not! Very occasionally, if somebody has only just developed diabetes, or has had a series of high glucose tests, puberty may be delayed slightly. Should this happen in your case, do not worry, everything will work properly eventually.

Remember that sexual intercourse is a form of exercise too – it is a well known and sometimes embarrassing cause of hypoglycaemia. Finally, there is no more reason why someone with diabetes should not form a permanent relationship or get married than someone without diabetes.

Is someone with diabetes normally fertile?

The answer is 'Yes', although, of course, there are exceptions. In the days before insulin was discovered, few women with diabetes conceived, and even fewer had live babies. It may still be true that a woman whose diabetes is very badly controlled might have some difficulty in conceiving, but where the condition is reasonably well controlled, conception should be normal.

Nor is there any reason why a healthy man with diabetes should not be able to father children. As with women, very badly controlled diabetes can temporarily lessen a man's fertility. Occasionally, diabetes can lead to male impotence, but this usually happens very much later in life.

Should a woman with diabetes have children?

Yes, if she wants to! She should normally be capable of bearing and caring for a child. However, should she have any serious complications – particularly complications involving the kidneys – the couple ought to think carefully before embarking on a pregnancy. If there are no complications, or only minor ones, then there should be no bar to pregnancy on account of the diabetes.

'Will our child get diabetes?'

This is perhaps the commonest question asked. The simple answer is 'No', because the likelihood of a baby being born with permanent diabetes is zero.

'But will my child develop diabetes, say at the age of five or ten?' Again, the answer is encouraging. The chances of your child developing diabetes in childhood, although greater than normal, are still small – something like 1 in 100 as opposed to the normal 1 in 500. By this reckoning, 99 out of every 100 children will not develop diabetes, and it would appear that most couples would consider this to be an acceptable risk.

You must remember that the answers to these questions are not certainties, they are only probabilities; one can never be sure that anyone will or will not get diabetes.

Some people ask whether there is any routine test that can predict whether their child will get diabetes. These are under development. Unfortunately they are too unreliable to give you a definite answer. Many children may show positive results on these tests but never get diabetes. This just causes a lot of unnecessary worry. They are therefore not recommended.

Children who get diabetes develop symptoms fairly quickly. If your child is unwell for any reason it is worth having a check for blood glucose. This is very easy to do. You should always ask your doctor if you are concerned about the possibility.

Diabetes and menstruation

Diabetes can have an effect on menstruation, particularly if the diabetes is poorly controlled. In such cases, periods may be upset, scanty, or missed altogether. But the most likely cause of a missed period is pregnancy!

Menstruation can have an effect on your diabetes. For instance, periods sometimes cause a variation in the blood glucose, and you may notice a definite change in the results of your blood or urine tests for a few days. If these changes are regular, there is no harm in increasing or decreasing your insulin dosage for a day or two, as indicated by your blood tests.

■ Pregnancy

A woman with diabetes needs special care before and during her pregnancy, and she should make every endeavour to keep her diabetes fully under control. In the past, about a third of the babies born to women with diabetes were lost. Now, with good care, the chances of losing a baby are only very slightly greater than for those women who do not have diabetes.

Before becoming pregnant

If you intend to start a family, or have another child, you should inform the doctor who helps you with your diabetes. This is necessary in case there are any medical problems that need dealing with before you become pregnant. Most importantly, you should obtain the best possible control of your diabetes. This is necessary to ensure that the newly conceived baby starts its development under the best possible conditions. The baby's organs are fully formed eight weeks after conception. The reason, therefore, for this special emphasis on good control before pregnancy is that babies are occasionally born with abnormalities. This is slightly more common in babies born to those with diabetes. If the glucose control is near perfect, then the chance of any of these abnormalities occurring is very small. (If the father has diabetes his control does not increase this risk.)

To achieve good standards of control it may be necessary to increase the number of injections. Certainly a minimum of two injections a day using mixtures of insulin will be required, and probably more frequent insulin injection will be necessary, especially as the pregnancy progresses.

Finally, it is now recommended that all women should take folic acid (one of the vitamins), if possible as soon as you start planning to have a baby and for the first 12 weeks of the pregnancy itself.

Control of diabetes during pregnancy

Keeping excellent control

Once pregnancy is confirmed, you should aim to achieve and maintain very good control. Fortunately, this becomes easier as the pregnancy proceeds. The aim is to achieve blood glucose levels between 4 and 7 mmol/l, before meals and less then 8 mmol/l afterwards. It is best for a pregnant woman to be cared for at a hospital with a special diabetic antenatal clinic. This allows you to meet with your diabetes specialist nurse, doctor, obstetrician and midwife together. During your pregnancy it will probably be necessary for you to visit the clinic every two to four weeks, in order that your diabetic control can be carefully monitored.

Monitoring your control

Frequent blood tests are important and must be performed carefully during pregnancy. Urine tests are of no value, because glucose often leaks into the urine rather more easily than usual during pregnancy. You will need to adjust the insulin, probably more often than normal, and this will only be possible with quite frequent testing. Occasionally poor control may mean that you are admitted to hospital for a few days, but this is the exception rather than the rule.

When you and your doctor are trying to get very tight control of your diabetes, there may be a slightly greater risk of hypoglycaemia than usual. This is especially likely in the early stages of pregnancy. This will cause your baby no harm.

Ketoacidosis, on the other hand, is damaging, but is almost entirely preventable. This is described in more detail elsewhere in the handbook (Chapter 7). Just remember that ketones develop when your fuel supply is below your needs, and this is aggravated if your insulin dosages are too low. Testing for ketones will be performed when you attend the clinic. But you may be advised to test yourself, especially if your blood glucose is running high (above 10 mmol/l). It is certainly wise to test for ketones if you are feeling unwell. If the tests are positive you will need to discuss this with your doctor.

Insulin dosage during pregnancy

Your insulin requirement is likely to increase during pregnancy, especially in the second half. Sometimes the dose goes up by 50–100 per cent or even more. However, you need not conclude that your diabetes is worse. The dose of insulin always falls to the pre-pregnancy amount as soon as the baby is born. As stated above, usually more than two injections of insulin a day are needed to ensure perfect control. Three or more injections using a pen device (similar to the regime described in Chapter 5) may be needed.

Diabetes developing during pregnancy

Occasionally, diabetes is discovered for the first time during pregnancy. This is usually detected as a result of a routine test which all pregnant women undergo. The initial treatment of this so-called 'gestational diabetes' is usually a change in the food that you eat. Occasionally, however, you may need insulin. In the majority of such cases the problem is resolved as soon as the baby has been delivered. If insulin treatment is started it is stopped after delivery and for those treated with diet no further treatment is required.

However, this type of diabetes is likely to recur with subsequent pregnancies. Any woman who has had this problem with her first child should always report to her doctor at once, if she thinks she is pregnant again.

Finally, a word of caution. If you have had 'gestational diabetes' you are somewhat more likely than average to develop the type of diabetes which occurs later in life. You would be advised to be careful with your weight and try to keep it as near normal as possible in order to help prevent this.

Monitoring your baby's growth

Your pregnancy will be supervised by the obstetric and diabetes teams working closely together. You may need to be seen every three to four weeks in the first part of the pregnancy and weekly or fortnightly in the later stages. Regular ultrasound tests will be performed to assess the baby's growth. These have to be done rather more often than in non-diabetic mothers. Sometimes additional tests may be necessary to assess the baby's heart rate, breathing and movements.

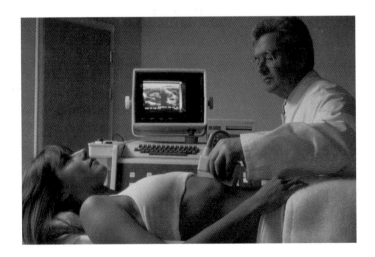

Ultrasound scan

Having your baby

Hospital admission

It is sometimes recommended that women with diabetes are admitted a week or so before their baby is due, so that a very careful check can be made on the diabetic control and on the baby's progress. Earlier delivery than normal is quite often recommended. This is because some babies born to women with diabetes are heavier than usual. If the mother goes the full 40 weeks, the size of her baby may make labour difficult. However, if tests of the baby's development show that it is quite normal and your diabetes control has been good, the pregnancy may be allowed to go to the full term before delivery, and you will be advised to come into hospital as soon as you go into labour. You should not normally deliver after your due date as the baby may then become too large and this can cause problems.

The method of delivery

The method of delivery will be influenced by many factors. Normal, vaginal delivery is preferable. If, however, a woman has previously had a Caesarean section, or the baby is large, shows any signs of distress during labour, or is the wrong way up (breech), then a Caesarean section is usually performed.

Controlling your diabetes during labour

During labour, at the stage when you are no longer able or advised to eat, an intravenous drip (a tube inserted in a vein in the arm) is nearly always set up. You will be given glucose and insulin through this tube using a special pump.

Blood glucose measurements will be carried out every hour or two, in order to check that your diabetes is being adequately controlled. Very soon after your baby has been born, the drip will be stopped, and insulin will be given by injection.

Remember, as soon as your baby is born you should go immediately on to the dose of insulin you were taking before the pregnancy started.

After the birth

The first few days

For the first few hours or days after the birth, the baby usually needs closer observation than normal and it may be necesary to do this in a special neonatal ward. This will be necessary if, for example:

■ The birth has been difficult
■ The baby is large.

In most cases, however, babies born to parents with diabetes are healthy from the start, and after the first few hours of observation there should be no reason why your baby should not be with you and be cared for in the same way as other newborn babies.

The first few weeks

Your baby may be born a little heavier than average, and his or her weight gain may be less in the first few weeks than expected. Indeed, some weight loss may occur, but don't be alarmed if this happens.

Summary

■ If you plan to become pregnant, try to balance your diabetes as well as possible.
■ Consult your doctor or clinic, preferably before you conceive and certainly as soon as you become pregnant.
■ Test regularly and carefully.
■ Adjust your insulin to achieve blood test results of 4 to 7 mmol/l.

Controlling your diabetes after you have had your baby

Controlling your diabetes when you get home from hospital will require a little more effort than it did before your baby was born.

Immediately after your baby has been delivered, your insulin requirements will fall. Therefore, the day following the birth you should return to the type and dose of insulin you were taking before you became pregnant. If you only started taking insulin during the pregnancy, the chances are that once your baby is born you can stop having injections altogether.

What about breast feeding?

There is no reason why you should not breast feed your baby, if you so choose. However, if you do breast feed, you will need to take extra carbohydrate at meals and snacks to compensate for loss of glucose in the breast milk. In addition, night feeds will mean that you are working harder. You must have your snacks regularly, and extra carbohydrate at night. Feed your baby and yourself at the same time.

Should blood tests be continued?

During your pregnancy you will almost certainly have achieved very good control of your blood glucose. Although blood testing need not be quite as frequent, it is sensible to keep this going. In this way risks to your own health will be kept to a minimum.

How many children should a woman with diabetes have?

There is no definite answer to this question. The need for extra care during pregnancy, and the need for admission to hospital towards the end of pregnancy, may be good reasons for restricting the size of the family. After two Caesarean sections, most obstetricians would advise against any more pregnancies. In the end, of course, the decision must rest with the parents.

Adoption

There is no particular reason why someone with Type 1, and who has no late complications, should not adopt a child. Adoption agencies do, however, require that prospective parents are fit and well, and that they have a responsible attitude to their health. Unfortunately very few babies are now available for adoption.

■ Contraception

Which type of contraceptive?

There are no forms of contraception which are forbidden, or known to be particularly harmful, to women with diabetes. None the less, some forms do seem to be slightly better than others.

The cap and sheath

Using these poses no problems.

Intrauterine devices

The 'coil' seems to be a satisfactory method of contraception for those with diabetes, though slightly less safe than the cap or sheath. In many women the coil has remained in position for a year or more, but there does appear to be a slightly greater risk of inflammation or infection in those with diabetes.

The 'pill'

The 'pill' is the most convenient form of contraceptive but is not suitable for everyone. Those with a raised blood pressure, or thrombosis, should not take the pill.

Generally speaking, there is little or no risk involved in a young woman taking the pill for short periods – say, a year or so. For longer term use, however, there is a slightly increased risk of accelerating blood vessel complications. For this reason it may be preferable to use the 'mini' or progesterone-only pill, the use of which appears not to carry such risks.

If you take the usual type of pill, which contains oestrogen, you may find that your blood glucose rises a little, so that you may need to adjust your insulin dose.

Sterilisation

Sterilisation in women, by tying the Fallopian tubes, or in men, by vasectomy, can be performed as easily and as safely in those with diabetes as in those without diabetes.

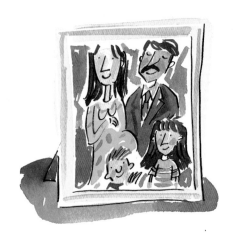

10 Diabetes in Children and Adolescents

Type 1 diabetes and its treatment have been fully described in previous chapters. The information presented there applies equally to children. The same balance should be aimed for, and the adjustments to diet, exercise and insulin are all similar. This chapter has been written to answer the questions asked by the parents of children with diabetes.

■ Childhood diabetes

You probably noticed how, after only a few injections, your son or daughter began to look and feel better. It is likely, however, that despite the feeling of relief that all is well, your original shock on hearing the diagnosis was followed by disbelief, anger, or even guilt that it might be your fault. First, it should be emphasised that there is nothing that you have done which has been responsible for the development of your child's diabetes. Diabetes is caused by damage to the beta cells of the pancreas and possibly by a virus or antibody, together with some genetic predisposition, and there is no way that you could have prevented this.

Once the blood glucose is controlled your child will lose all his or her symptoms. Growth and development should be entirely normal. These will be assessed regularly. There should be very little limitation on activities, school life, sport, etc.

■ Diabetes and small children

Insulin injections

Problems faced by parents

One of the most heartbreaking prospects for parents is having to give their child injections. However, once you have given your child his or her injection for the first time, you will know that it is not as frightening as you imagined. But what about your child?

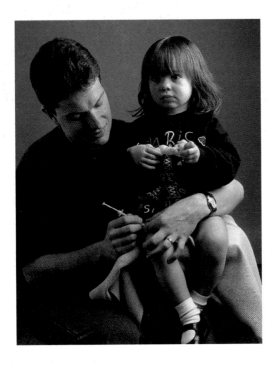

Parents quickly learn the technique of injecting insulin

For infants and very young children, it is difficult to explain why injections are necessary. All parents find their own way of coping. You will be no exception. If there is a secret to success, it is a consistent approach. Attempts to deceive or encourage with false promises that there will be only a few more injections are best avoided. Distraction and/or relaxation techniques may help – advice on these should be available from your specialist nurse. You will quickly learn that patience, persistence and understanding are the qualities most essential to the parents of a child with diabetes. Parents may find it helpful to join a parents' or self-help group. If you contact Diabetes UK they will be able to tell you whether a group of this sort exists in your area. All family members can help – it should not just be left to mum.

At what age should children inject themselves?

There is no set age by which children must be able to inject themselves, but, ideally, they should all be doing so by the time they move from primary to secondary school.

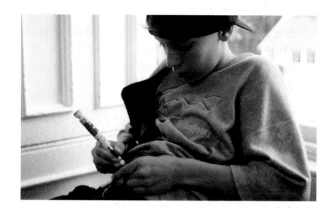

Many children over the age of six can do their own injections

If your child shows the slightest inclination towards carrying out all or part of the injection or testing procedure, do encourage them from the start and reward them for doing so. For example, they could choose a site or push the plunger. Many children over the age of five or six can give their injections quite easily. It is wise for you to check the dose and that it is correctly drawn up, however. Most children consider injecting themselves to be less painful than being injected by their parents, and when they have given their first injection, they are proud of their achievement. They may often choose to continue giving them all. Whenever your child starts to take over, parents should continue for some while to keep an eye on them.

Injection sites and technique

It is as important to inject insulin correctly as it is to measure the dose. Most children, if they are old enough to give their own injections, quickly learn the technique and do it well for the first few months. Then they may discover that injections are less painful if they always inject in exactly the same place. Unfortunately, repeated injections at the same site will eventually damage the skin and underlying tissues. This can cause an unsightly lump (called lipohypertrophy). But worse than the appearance is the fact that insulin injected into the lump may not be absorbed properly. Control may become sufficiently poor to persuade the unsuspecting parents to increase the dose of insulin. If, on a later occasion, the child tries a new injection site, the larger dose of insulin will be absorbed properly and may cause a hypoglycaemic reaction.

Injections can be given in the thighs, buttocks, abdominal wall and arms. Usually insulin is absorbed (and therefore works) more quickly when injected into the abdomen as opposed to the thigh. For consistency it is suggested that one site should be used for the morning injection and another site used for the evening injection. Injections can be switched from one side to the other on alternate days (see page 39). Children should use the shorter needle – 5 or 8 mm – not the adult 12.7 mm

Syringes, pens and other aids

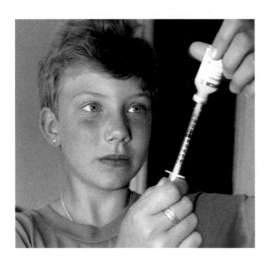

The standard syringe is easy to use and handle. Pen devices are available which are found by many to be more convenient. These contain a cartridge of insulin (thus avoiding the drawing up procedure). They can be carried in a pocket and used whenever needed. The cartridge usually contains enough insulin for several days.

Problems of hypoglycaemia in small children

The effects of hypoglycaemic reactions in children

A major fear of most parents with a small child with diabetes is that hypoglycaemia might go unrecognised. People are afraid that the child could then lapse into a coma, perhaps leading to brain damage. If you have a very young child your concern could be even greater. You may think that your child will not recognise the symptoms or will fail to tell you about them. These fears are usually unwarranted. The symptoms of hypoglycaemia are usually quite obvious. If they should occur at night the child almost invariably wakes up. Death due to hypoglycaemia occurs only extremely rarely. Brain damage occurs only under very exceptional circumstances.

These problems do not occur for the following reason. As the hypoglycaemic reaction occurs, the body senses that the blood glucose is too low and corrective mechanisms are started: first, the breaking down of body stores of glucose; second, the production of a substance called glucagon. This hormone stimulates the blood glucose to rise – ultimately back to normal.

Why, then, does the hypoglycaemic reaction occur? The answer is simply that the body's response is not fast enough. However, it will catch up eventually and the child will recover completely, even if no sugar has been given. Hypoglycaemic reactions should only cause serious concern when severe reactions (ie causing unconsciousness) are occurring frequently.

Small children especially tend to be more prone to hypoglycaemia than adults. This is because their range of physical activity and the amount they eat at mealtimes may vary very much more. For this reason we suggest the ideal blood sugar to aim for in those under five may be 5–10 mmol/l as opposed to the 4–8 mmol/l target suggested in previous chapters.

Hypoglycaemic reaction and convulsions

Occasionally, because of the rapid lowering of blood glucose during hypoglycaemia, the brain may respond by producing a convulsion (commonly called a 'fit'). This is one of the most frightening aspects of hypoglycaemia. However, if you have experienced someone suffering a convulsion, you will know that the effects appear much more alarming than they really are. The convulsions are sometimes incorrectly termed 'epileptic fits'. The type of convulsion is similar to that seen in epilepsy, but it does not mean that your child is developing this condition as well.

What should you do if your child has a convulsion? First, if your child is unconscious or having a fit, you should not try to get him or her to take anything by mouth. In any case, this may be virtually impossible to do, since the teeth may be tightly clenched. Within a few minutes, however, the body will start to produce glucose from its own stores, the blood glucose will rise and your child will recover. Thus, although it may seem very frightening when this first happens, you can be reassured that all will be well within a few minutes.

Hypoglycaemia at night

One of the major fears of parents is hypoglycaemia at night. As indicated above, even if hypoglycaemia is observed your child will recover spontaneously with time. Usually, however, children wake up, or with severe hypoglycaemia, eg with convulsions, will wake you.

There is no reason to worry unduly and certainly there is no need to set up a night rota so that your child is constantly watched over.

However, you will want to avoid night hypoglycaemia if possible. Adjustment of the type and dose of insulin in the evening can, especially with modern very quick-acting insulin, enable them to be avoided (see Chapter 7, 'Night hypoglycaemia', page 120).

Treatment of severe reactions

Obviously, severe reactions are best avoided whenever possible, but if they should occur, Hypostop can be tried as long as the child is able to swallow. If this does not work, they can be dealt with by means of a simple injection with the hormone glucagon.

Glucagon is available on prescription, in the form of a simple kit. It should be injected either under the skin or into a muscle (see page 118). Do not give the whole vial to a child – approximately one-third to a half is usually enough. Within a few minutes the unconscious child should recover – but as the effect of glucagon is only temporary you must always give some carbohydrate once consciousness has been regained. If recovery does not occur, then you should call a doctor immediately.

Here are the steps you must take if your child has a convulsion or is deeply unconscious:

- Lie your child down on his/her side.
- Keep him/her warm.
- Do not try to give sugar or sugar fluid.
- Give an injection of glucagon.
- Once recovery takes place, give a glass of water or juice with two to four teaspoonsful of sugar.
- If recovery does not occur, or if this is the first time that your child has had a convulsion, call your doctor. If your child is still unconscious when he arrives, he can easily give glucose into a vein, which works in a few seconds.
- Sometimes if glucagon is given vomiting may occur for a short while afterwards.
- Finally, it is worth testing the blood glucose a little while after recovery. If it falls again you may need to give more sugar-containing fluids.

Is it a hypoglycaemic reaction?

When your child looks peaky or is unwell, you may be unsure as to whether these symptoms are due to a hypoglycaemic reaction. A headache can be an indication of hypoglycaemia, especially if it occurs in the early morning. Variation in mood is also sometimes caused by low blood glucose. If this is the case it should not last long and will rapidly improve with sugar. In most cases where these odd symptoms occur your child will not be hypoglycaemic – but, of course, you will want to be sure. You will quite quickly get to know the pattern of your child's hypoglycaemic reactions. However, with small children whose behaviour and health wax and wane with remarkable speed, you may find it more difficult to decide. The only foolproof way of finding out is to perform a blood test.

Understandably, you may not want to perform blood tests every time your child is below par. The best guide as to what you should do is the timing of the reactions. If they are occurring at a time when you would expect your child to be hungry or short of glucose, give him or her something to eat. You need only be concerned if these episodes happen very frequently. If you are constantly having to provide a lot of extra carbohydrate, or your child is getting fat, a different strategy may be needed. Most children will quickly realise that if they say that they 'feel funny', they may get a chocolate bar – and who would not exploit this possibility!

If blood tests are normal or high (4 or greater) when these episodes occur, then your child is not suffering a hypoglycaemic reaction.

What about the next dose of insulin after a hypoglycaemic reaction?

After a reaction occurs, especially if it happens just before the next insulin injection, you may well worry what to do. Should the next injection be given? The answer is always 'yes'. Once your child has recovered, the insulin must be given normally in the normal dose. Remember, it was the previous dose that caused the reaction. If you reduce or omit the dose the blood glucose may become very high. This may be a lot worse for the body than a hypoglycaemic reaction.

If, however, your child has had a cluster of reactions causing unconsciousness, say two or three in a week, it is worth just reducing the dosages of insulin for a few days, allowing the blood glucose to run a little on the high side. The reason for this is that after a bad reaction sometimes the warning system in the body gets slightly blunted, which is why several may occur without warning in a cluster. By allowing the blood glucose to run a little high for a couple of days, the system is restored to normal.

Intelligence and hypoglycaemic reactions

Many parents worry that episodes of hypoglycaemia, especially if associated with bouts of unconsciousness or convulsions, may lead to deterioration in the intelligence and development of their child. Mild hypoglycaemia has no effect on growth or mental development, and neither does occasional severe hypoglycaemia. Repeated severe hypoglycaemia, for example, with convulsions should be avoided in those under seven.

Problems with food

Too much ... too little

If your child seems constantly hungry, then it would be appropriate, as with any other child, to give him or her more to eat. Unless you are sure that the hunger is due to a reaction, any additional food should be given at normal meal and snack times. If your child is of normal weight, there is no harm in increasing the amount of food, but if your child is overweight or fat, then some care is necessary in giving anything extra. Remember that it is normal for a child's appetite to increase with age. Refer to your dietitian for specific advice on diet.

Never reduce the recommended diet

IMPORTANT: if blood glucose levels are higher than normal, you must NEVER try to improve your child's diabetic control by cutting down on food or cutting out normal meals.

Should your child be getting a supply of sugar, in the form of sweets or sweet drinks, without your consent, this ought to be prevented, but your child's normal diet should not be reduced in an attempt to improve the results of the tests. If the blood tests are high with a normal diet, your child needs more insulin, not less food. Again, if you are at all concerned about your child's diet, you should speak to your local dietitian.

Parties

As far as possible, your child's social activities should continue as normal. With smaller children you may worry about what they might eat when not under your supervision. Party foods may not be those that you would normally choose. Eaten occasionally they will not be a problem. Generally speaking, children do not eat excessively at parties. Even if they do this is often balanced by an increase in activity. The worst that might happen is a rise in tests for a day or two, but this will do no harm.

You may be concerned about the timing of the teatime insulin injection. If the party is during the afternoon, it is probably best to give the injection when your child comes home, with a top-up snack before bedtime. If the party is prolonged into the evening, then it is best to give the injection before the party meal, if it is not too complicated to arrange.

More information on parties and discos is given on pages 202 and 203.

If children would prefer to have their evening injection away from home, this may be much easier using one of the pen devices, which can be easily carried and used.

Problems with tests

Small children and testing

With very small children and infants, testing may be a problem. Blood tests can, of course, be performed by you but you will probably want to avoid pricking your small child too often. If you feel that your child is unwell and you are concerned as to whether the blood glucose might be too high or too low, there is no alternative, but for routine monitoring urine tests may be quite helpful. Once your child is potty trained urine testing is straightforward. Problems can arise, however, with a child who is still in nappies, although simply squeezing a little urine from a wet nappy onto a testing strip may be adequate.

With all children, but especially the younger ones, it is difficult to get them to urinate at exactly the time you need to perform a test. In such cases, just make a note of the times that urine is passed and your doctor can then help you to interpret the results of these tests, so that you can make any necessary adjustments to your child's diet or insulin dose. However, if you and your child will tolerate it, blood tests tend to be more reliable and helpful in enabling you to check that insulin dosages are correct.

'Why must I be tested?'

This question is often asked by children. Although many youngsters can appreciate the reasons for testing, the very young cannot be expected to understand what is being done or why. Even so, most children become so accustomed to tests, that they view them in much the same way as any of their other routines, such as brushing their teeth and washing. Young children question the reasons less frequently than older children, who often do not want to accept the inconvenience of what they consider to be a boring routine.

Frequently, older children may practise all sorts of ploys to avoid tests: 'My tests were all normal, so I haven't written them down', 'I forgot' or 'I threw it (the urine) away by mistake'. In dealing with this situation bribery is unwise. You should adopt a consistent approach in which you reinforce the message that tests are essential if treatment is to be balanced and health and fitness maintained.

Insulin adjustment

More insulin

When tests are consistently high, ie above 10, more insulin is required. At such times, parents frequently ask, 'Can I adjust the insulin dose myself?' The answer to this question is 'Yes'. In fact, an adjustment of insulin should be the rule, rather than the exception. Adjustment of insulin dosage during growth spurts and puberty is normal and necessary. Of course, during the early stages you will need advice from your doctor, specialist nurse or diabetes health visitor as to when and by how much the insulin dose should be increased. There are no set rules, because the dose required by each child is different. More insulin is often required when your child is less active, for example when at home for the weekend, or on holiday, or during any of the childhood illnesses.

Less insulin

If your child suffers frequent reactions (especially if they occur at approximately the same time of day), less insulin may be needed.

Giving less insulin is preferable to attempting to counter persistent reactions by giving excess glucose or sweet things. By getting to know how long the effect of each insulin dose lasts, you should be able to work out which dose or type of insulin should be reduced and by how much.

Children often require less insulin when they are at school, since at such times they may be more active and consequently their blood glucose is lower.

Initially, adjusting the insulin dose will undoubtedly seem frighteningly complicated. However with practice and guidance from doctors and diabetes specialist nurses you will soon become quite capable of making the necessary adjustments.

- The child with a high blood glucose needs more insulin.
- The child with a low blood glucose needs less insulin or more food.

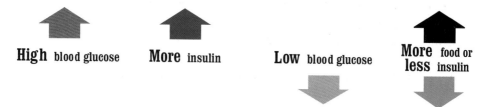

As for making a major error and causing damage to your child, if you make the sort of adjustments you have been advised, then the risks are negligible.

When you have to be away from your child

There will be occasions when you wish to leave your child in the care of somebody else. A close relative will probably be aware of how to take care of your child, but a babysitter will need some simple instructions.

■ School and diabetes

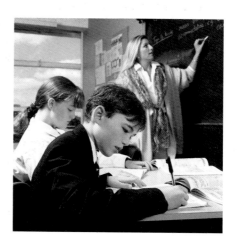

Telling the teacher

It is important that all the teachers that deal with your child are aware that he or she has diabetes, for two reasons:

1. Mid-morning or afternoon snacks must be permitted and, particularly in the case of young children, the teachers can help to ensure that these and main meals are taken on time and not missed.

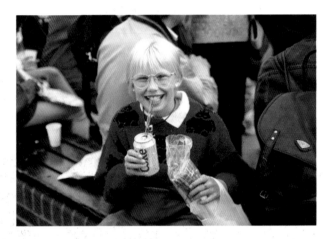

2. The teachers should understand what is happening if your child has a hypoglycaemic reaction. Teachers should be told how to treat these reactions, and should be discouraged from sending your child home, when giving a biscuit or two or three lumps of sugar or glucose tablets is sufficient to curtail most reactions.

Unnecessary fear of reactions and overprotective attitudes will be prevented by having discussions with the teachers as soon as your child starts school, or when diabetes is first diagnosed.

Your specialist nurse or doctor will be pleased to visit the school and discuss your child's diabetes with the teacher if you wish. You could give them a copy of the special information sheet for teachers available from Diabetes UK. This provides advice to help them if problems should arise.

Hypo treatment at school

Teachers must be encouraged not to be frightened by hypoglycaemic reactions. Alongside advice that hypos are rapidly corrected by taking something sweet, it is a good idea for the class teacher to be given a small container of short- and long-acting carbohydrates. We suggest a supply of:

- Glucose tablets
- Ordinary (not low calorie) fizzy drinks or small bottles of Lucozade
- Biscuits such as ginger nuts, oat or garibaldis
- Cereal bars.

Some parents like the school to have a supply of Hypostop.

School meals

Parents often worry about the quality and quantity of school meals. The choice lies between school dinners, packed lunches, and coming home for lunch. It is important that your child should do as other children do, and not be made to feel or appear different in any way.

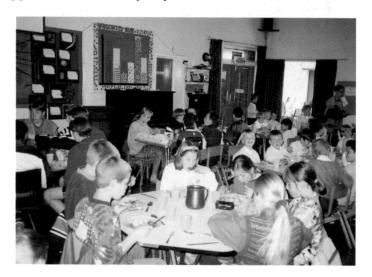

School meals usually contain adequate amounts of carbohydrate to provide the correct balance. You should not be overconcerned that mistakes may be made which will upset your child's diabetic control. If the school operates a cafeteria system, it may be more difficult for your child to select the right type of food, although it may prove to be a valuable learning experience. If your child is very young, you can check through the school menus, and ask the teacher concerned to help with the right choice of food.

The decision as to whether or not your child should have school meals should not be influenced by their diabetes.

A lot of worry is sometimes caused when teachers report that a child does not eat their school meal or packed lunch, or on occasions gives their packed lunch to a friend. The concern, obviously, is that the child might develop hypoglycaemia. However, with smallish children appetite is an important factor. If their blood glucose levels are falling, their appetite is likely to increase and they will eat what is needed. If their appetite is blunted and they do not actually want the meal, it is probably unlikely that they will go hypoglycaemic.

Exercise

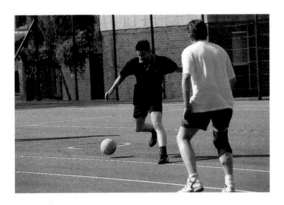

Exercise and sport are essential for all children with diabetes

At school, the timing and extent of exercise can usually be determined in advance and any difficulties anticipated. Below, we answer some of the questions parents most commonly ask about exercise.

> Do I need to give my child extra carbohydrate before exercise?

Yes. It is essential that games teachers appreciate the importance of this extra carbohydrate, and ensure that your child takes it before any exercise.

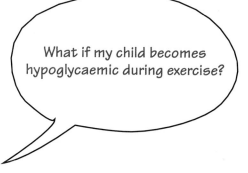

Are there any activities or sports in which my child should not participate?

No, having diabetes is no bar to participating in any normal sporting activity, and it should not be used as an excuse for missing games. Very high levels of achievement have been reached in many sports by those with diabetes.

Older children may wish to take part in more dangerous sports, such as climbing or sailing, and these activities need to be given more careful consideration. It is essential that your child should be accompanied, and that hypoglycaemic reactions are prevented. Basically, children with and without diabetes need similar supervision in such sports. However, those supervising the sports should be advised about the symptoms and treatment of hypoglycaemia.

What if my child becomes hypoglycaemic during exercise?

Your child should take more sugar. Make sure the teachers in charge know exactly what to do. It is helpful for children to wear games clothes with pockets, especially for sports like cross-country running, so that if they should become shaky they have sugar on them and can take some immediately.

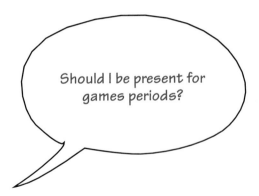

Should I be present for
games periods?

No. You should resist any pressure which might be exerted to
persuade you to be present, since this would merely serve to single
out your child as being 'different'.

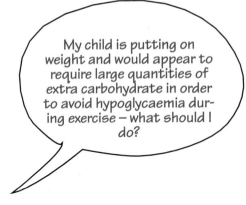

My child is putting on
weight and would appear to
require large quantities of
extra carbohydrate in order
to avoid hypoglycaemia during exercise – what should I
do?

The best advice is to reduce the insulin dosage, rather than continue
to increase the carbohydrate intake. This should be done on the days
when heavy exercise is likely, with a return to the normal insulin
dosage on other days.

If hypos do occur use pure carbohydrate such as glucose tablets rather
than chocolate or chocolate bars which may contain a lot of fat.

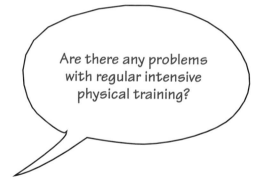

How should I deal with
unexpected periods of
exercise, say at weekends

On most occasions an extra portion or two of carbohydrate will be
sufficient to guard against any risk of hypoglycaemia.

Are there any problems
with regular intensive
physical training?

Many children, especially older ones, who get involved in
competitive sports want to undertake regular and arduous
physical training. This in itself poses no problems and the
precautions taken for any other exercise should be undertaken.
However, with very hard physical training the effects on the body
may be prolonged and hypoglycaemic reactions may occur several
hours later. Since these training programmes often take place in
the evening, this may lead to a reaction during the night. Sometimes the blood sugar rises after exercise – this occurs when
inadequate insulin is present. Care is required before very
strenuous exercise if the blood sugar is already high, and especially
if your child is unwell. Exercise may make this worse and very
heavy exercise is best avoided (see page 192).

I get very worried when my child goes off to play alone or with friends at the local recreation ground – should I take any special precautions?

This is a cause of concern for many parents. The guiding principle should be to provide the same supervision for a child with diabetes as you would for any other child of the same age. If your child has a mishap, whether it be a broken ankle or a hypoglycaemic reaction, friends will always summon aid, so don't worry unduly!

The effect of stress on diabetes

One of the commonest reasons for an increase in blood glucose is anxiety. All children are stressed at times; it may be minor worries about losing something, or failing to complete work to the teacher's satisfaction. In those without diabetes, these stresses may go unnoticed, but with diabetes they may be revealed by high blood glucose levels. If you are perplexed by inexplicable changes in the control pattern, stress could well be the answer.

Occasionally, severe stress may be associated with hypoglycaemia, especially in small children. It is, however, more common for the blood glucose to rise.

Testing at school

It is clearly awkward for children to perform tests at school. However, unlike urine tests, blood tests can be performed in public, though some children may be shy about this. Luckily, with modern devices these have become easier to do. For many children, however, the midday test may not be absolutely essential and, if control is otherwise good, can be avoided. If your child is having difficulty with control, there is a choice of blood testing or dipstick urine testing, which may give you information about the blood glucose while they are at school.

School attendance and performance

School attendance should be the same as for any other child. In general, it is found that children with diabetes are not absent from school significantly more than their non-diabetic counterparts.

Your child's intellectual, sporting and general activities should also be similar to those of other children.

Staying away, holidays and travel

Children with diabetes should be encouraged to participate in all those activities which would be expected of other children. These include nights or weekends away, camps of various kinds, and travel at home and overseas. Certainly, you should not discourage your child from going on holiday either in this country or abroad.

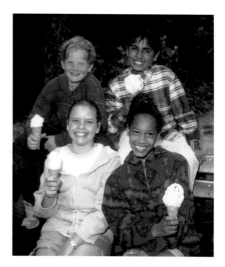

Nights and weekends away

All parents are apprehensive the first time their child stays away from home. However, as the parent of a child with diabetes you will feel particularly concerned. Before your son or daughter stays away you should be sure that:

1. Your child is capable of giving his or her own injections, or there is an adult present who can give them.

2. The people with whom your child will be staying are fully aware of the possibility of hypoglycaemic reactions, and know what to do should they face one. You should not be afraid to ask them to:

    ■ Be particularly attentive to any changes in your child's moods or health.
    ■ Make sure the diet does not contain excessively sweet food.
    ■ Check that insulin is taken at the correct dosage and at the set times.

■ Remember that sometimes reactions can occur for no very obvious reason and are not the fault of the person looking after the child.

■ If they have concerns about these points, then your diabetes specialist nurse can liaise with them and reassure them.

You will find that most responsible people will be only too willing to help in any way possible. Whenever you feel anxious, always remind yourself that even untreated children will recover from reactions.

Camps

Cub camps, Brownie weekends and brigade camps are important childhood activities. They are always well supervised by people with first aid experience, and as long as you inform them about your child's diabetes, you may be confident that all will be well.

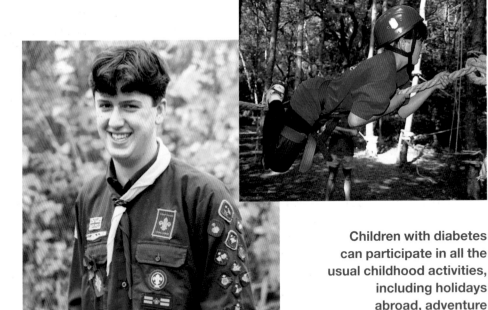

Children with diabetes can participate in all the usual childhood activities, including holidays abroad, adventure holidays and camps

For children worried by the prospect of going away from home, Diabetes UK's educational holidays perform a very important function, enabling them to enjoy a holiday in a situation where they need not feel the 'odd person out'. Because the camps are well supervised by specialist staff, you should be able to feel at ease in the knowledge that your child is being provided with the best possible care. More of these are also being organised on a local basis, so your child will not be too far from home. For more information, contact Diabetes UK.

Travel

Effects of travel

Overseas travel should pose no particular problems. Your experience of selecting the right sort of food for your child when at home will enable you to select from even the most unusual foreign menus. The worst that can happen is that the blood glucose level goes a little higher than normal.

Travel sickness

The journey itself usually has little influence on the diabetes, apart from travel sickness. Although this is relatively common, you may worry that vomiting may lead to diabetic ketoacidosis (see page 109). Fortunately, travel sickness is confined to the period of travel, and as soon as the motion ceases, so do the nausea and vomiting. With long car journeys, break the journey frequently, avoid reading and, if necessary, try to obtain some motion sickness tablets from your doctor. Should your child be sick, give sweetened juices every hour to ensure that loss of fluid and fat breakdown do not occur. If you are on a long journey, say by sea, you may find that glucose levels may rise, in which case an increase in insulin may be necessary.

Meal times

Most children find journeys exciting, and hence it is likely that the blood glucose will rise. Therefore, hypoglycaemic reactions during long journeys are most unlikely, and you should keep snacks and meals as near to normal times as possible. Increasing the food intake should not be necessary, but it is a wise precaution to carry some extra snacks, in case meals should be unduly delayed.

When travelling by car make sure that the snacks are easily accessible and not in the boot.

Air travel

Air travel can be a little difficult due to time changes. This subject is discussed in more detail in on pages 196 to 202.

Insurance

When travelling abroad you should always make sure that you have some health insurance (see page 189), and in an EU country you should have the appropriate forms for free treatment (Form E111), available from your local DSS office.

Vaccination and immunisation

Vaccinations and immunisations can be given to your child in exactly the same way as to any other child. The worst that can happen is that with some types of vaccination, such as that for typhoid, your child may feel slightly unwell for 24 hours or so, and that the blood glucose may rise. If this happens, you may need to increase the dose of insulin, just as you would with any other minor illness.

Sickness while away

Short vomiting illnesses are quite common. When travelling, these should be managed in exactly the same way as any other illness, and you should refer to pages 173 and 194. Familiarise yourself with these sections before you go on holiday.

Change in environment and activity

Undoubtedly children may be very much more active when away on holiday. In hot weather the effect of insulin is more pronounced – some reduction in dose may be necessary. Excitement in small children also tends to reduce the blood sugars. Finally, guides obtainable from Diabetes UK may be helpful for foreign travel.

■ Older children with diabetes

Teaching your child about diabetes

The earlier that children take some interest in their diabetes, particularly in giving their own injections, the better it is. They have to progress at their own pace. Pushing too hard may be counterproductive. In the early stages in younger children, detailed explanations are unlikely to be fully understood. However, as children grow older, it will be necessary for them to take complete command of their treatment, so that they can achieve the independence they seek. Their success depends, to a large extent, on you. Your child will need to learn as much about diabetes as you know, and be persuaded that the steps necessary to maintain good balance are worthwhile, because they ensure a fit, healthy, active life.

■ Adolescence

Adolescence, meaning 'to grow to maturity', is a relatively new concept first used during the nineteenth century. Society determines the nature, roles and expectations of adolescence. However, it is generally regarded as potentially a difficult time both for those going through it and for their parents.

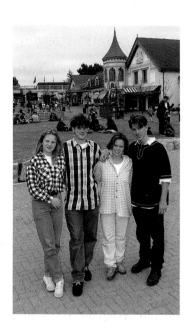

During adolescence physical and psychological changes occur that have implications for the person with diabetes.

Physical

Adolescence is a period of rapid growth and sexual development. There is increased resistance caused by the increase in growth hormone production, thus insulin doses increase. As growth hormone is produced mainly overnight this may be particularly noticeable first thing in the morning, the so-called 'dawn phenomenon', where blood sugars may increase. This is sometimes associated with hypoglycaemia in the early part of the night, especially when attempts are made to correct the morning test by increasing the previous evening's insulin dose. Ways of dealing with this are described under the section 'Night hypoglycaemia' in Chapter 7.

Psychological

The adolescent is striving to establish a sense of identity and is seeking independence from parents. It is also a time when peer group relationships strengthen and body image becomes all important.

This stage of development can lead to resentment, rejection of authority and high-risk behaviour. Diabetes management complicates matters further by expecting commitment and routine. It can lead to frustration and rejection of the diabetes regimen which is characterised by poor glycaemic control.

Educational

If diabetes is diagnosed early in life, ie at age 10 or earlier, most of the information or education is provided by the parent. As the child grows and develops, the parents obviously hope to transmit this information and education to the child, but this process is not always complete and very often parents, physicians and specialists may not recognise that a young adolescent does not have all the information they need. This is especially tough as life changes so quickly during adolescence in terms of increased activity and social life, etc. For this reason it is a good idea for the adolescent to have individual sessions of education to go through all the details necessary for self-care of diabetes with their diabetes specialist nurse. These can be of real value in providing answers to questions which you may not be able to answer adequately. They also serve the important function of reinforcing what you, as mum or dad, might have said – and as you will be only too aware, what mum or dad says is not always listened to!

Coping strategies

Parents

It is important that parents have an appreciation of both the physical and psychological changes during adolescence. Good two-way communication is to be encouraged, whilst there should be a gradual change in care provision – from providing care to supporting self-care. Parental involvement and support are vital during the adolescent years.

Health professionals

The health professionals should provide individualised holistic care. Education should be ongoing and incorporate aspects relevant to adolescent development. The relationship between professional and adolescent should be one of co-operation and encouragement of the individual in self-control.

Letting go

The most difficult decision encountered by parents of all adolescent children, whether they have diabetes or not, is when to let them take more control of their own lives. This is particularly difficult with young people with diabetes, where you will feel concern that, if your child is solely responsible for his or her tests and insulin injections and adjustment, they may make a mess of it. However, it is important that your child learns that they have to take charge of their own diabetes sooner or later. The best policy is to encourage your child, whenever possible, to do what they can and try to keep a discreet distance. Remember, if your child looks and behaves normally, he or she will not be coming to any immediate harm. Relatively short periods of high blood glucose, even lasting a few months, will not have serious consequences.

Ignoring diabetes

Most parents find that the adolescent may be more concerned about things other than their diabetes! They find the whole subject of diabetes boring, and the non-stop treatment tedious. As a result, fewer tests may be performed, and a degree of sloppiness may creep into insulin technique and the timing of doses. A lax attitude may develop with regard to the regularity of meals and the type of food eaten. It is as well for you to be prepared for this, otherwise it can cause considerable frustration and anger.

Try to appreciate that your child will be seeing himself or herself as an individual for the first time – an image that is marred by a total dependence on the daily injection of insulin. At a time when striving for independence is the main goal, many adolescents find this intolerable, and occasional displays of anger and rejection are hardly surprising. This period of rejection is, however, usually short-lived. It is important for you to remind yourself during this difficult time that short periods of loss of control – weeks or even a month or two – will not be serious in terms of its influence on long-term complications. Remain confident that your son or daughter will return to a more responsible approach to diabetes, and make every effort to:

- Try to be understanding.
- Treat your son or daughter as an adult rather than a child.

- ■ Encourage an attitude of responsibility with regard to treatment and clinic attendance.

- ■ Stay cool.

- ■ Finally, remember children and young teenagers worry about today or tomorrow. Threats about long-term complications are pointless!

Manipulation

Young people frequently develop ways of ensuring that their diabetes gives rise to as little inconvenience as possible. They work out that good blood tests are always approved of, and they may decide that the easiest way of achieving this is not to test at all, but simply to write down the desired results. Your doctor may perceive what is happening, but if they do not and you do, you should tell them, so that they can make sure that your child is getting the correct dose of insulin.

Children who have severe anxieties about their diabetes, or those who feel very insecure, may occasionally manipulate things in a more extreme and possibly risky way. For example, in an effort to get attention, they may even manipulate their insulin injections or meals so that reactions occur more frequently. This, of course, creates a good deal of concern from both parents and doctors, and may lead to admission to hospital, where the child will feel more secure. If your child shows signs of behaving in this disturbing way, you should seek expert help. You should not automatically feel that you are failing in some way to provide the care and support that your child needs. Also, you should remember that it is sometimes very difficult for children to express their fears about their health to anyone, perhaps least of all to their parents, whose esteem they treasure most highly. Sometimes, by causing reactions, they hope to get the help and attention of a third party, such as the doctor or specialist nurse, with whom they may be able to discuss their problems more readily.

Of major concern, however, is if you notice that your child – more usually a girl – is trying to lose weight, and despite eating much less than normal is running high blood sugars. This is especially serious if she is reducing her insulin. Some may learn that this results in loss of weight. However, this must be taken seriously as it may be an indication of an eating disorder ('anorexia'). Expert advice is needed to detect this early and provide treatment.

Teenage activities

As your child grows up, his or her activities will become very much more varied. Some routines, which were once easy, often become more difficult to maintain. Therefore, it is important that diabetes should impose as few restrictions as possible on day-to-day activities. A greater frequency of insulin injections provides considerably more flexibility, thereby enabling the time of, say, the evening meal, to be changed in order to permit participation in after-school activities. If the evening meal is delayed by more than half an hour, a small snack should be eaten to cover any residual effects of the previous insulin dose. The evening dose of insulin should then be given before the main meal.

Parties, discos, etc

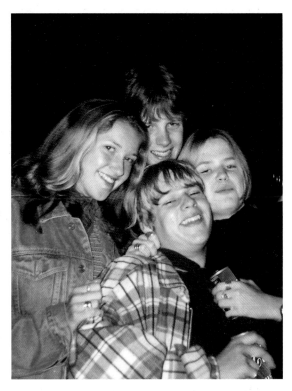

Advice about adjusting insulin and food to cope with parties and discos is given on pages 202 to 203.

One other aspect of teenage life which may worry you is that your child might eat the wrong sort of food and drink sucrose-containing drinks when at parties or discos. If this happens it is not going to cause any major problems, so don't worry unnecessarily. It is vital that your child should not be constantly precluded from normal teenage activities, simply because of his or her diabetes.

Alcohol

As described on page 67, there is no doubt that alcohol can affect the blood glucose. It usually causes a fall in blood glucose and therefore may contribute to a hypoglycaemic reaction. However, the majority of people with diabetes who wish to take alcohol, learn to cope with it perfectly well, provided it is not to excess. It is probably wise, however, to experiment a bit in a safe environment, such as the home, with small amounts of alcohol to see what effect it has on the blood glucose. One individual varies a great deal from another. However, all young people should be advised that, if they are going to take alcohol, they must be careful to make sure they have plenty to eat, and that the blood glucose is more likely to go down than up; finally, that they need to avoid getting drunk as this and hypoglycaemia can be a dangerous combination.

Finally beware of drugs – some can be very dangerous, especially for those with diabetes. Cannabis may accentuate or mask hypoglycaemia. Ecstasy is known to cause sudden death or precipitate ketoacidosis.

Job selection

During teenage life your children will be making decisions about what jobs they should undertake. It is wise to emphasise to them fairly early on that, unfortunately, there are certain jobs which they cannot do for legal reasons. It should be stressed that this is due not to any deficiency on their part, but to problems that might occur with hypoglycaemic reactions and cause dangers to others. These jobs include those in the Armed Forces, Police, or driving public service or heavy goods vehicles. This means that the vast majority of jobs are open to everybody with diabetes and diabetes should prove no barrier to them. Remember that your local diabetes physician or specialist nurse may well be able to provide support and references if you are worried that some discrimination may be involved.

Sex

Fortunately sexual life is unimpaired by diabetes in young people. The sorts of problems that may occur after very many years of diabetes, which sometimes affect potency, do not apply. If your male children have read about this, they can be completely reassured. Like any other form of exercise, making love may be associated with hypoglycaemia and this can be a cause of embarrassment. This may be avoided by taking the same steps as for other forms of exercise. In girls, especially if diagnosed at around the age of 10 to 13, diabetes may cause some disturbance in menstrual function. Periods may be delayed for a few months or up to a year, but almost always sort themselves out once control of the diabetes is achieved.

Fertility in young women is unaffected by diabetes. Contraception can and should be used as soon as appropriate.

■ Children with diabetes and other illnesses

The effect of diabetes on other illnesses and their treatment

Many parents are concerned that diabetes may lead to increased frequency of other illnesses. The fears are, in the main, groundless, and your child should be no more prone to catching coughs, colds and childhood infections, such as chickenpox, than any other child.

A child with diabetes can undergo all forms of treatment. With operations, however, one or two special precautions will need to be taken. For example, if the operation is likely to lead to a long period during which your child is unable to eat, then a drip or intravenous feeding may be necessary.

Dentistry

Some precautions are necessary to maintain diabetic balance during treatment. Further details are provided on page 136.

Can other illnesses affect your child's diabetes?

Yes, any illness will tend to raise the blood glucose, requiring an increase in the insulin dose.

Particular care is required with illnesses associated with:

■ Vomiting

■ Nausea

■ Loss of appetite.

These are far more common in children than in adults, and vomiting, in particular, can be associated with almost any illness. The standard procedures to be followed in cases of vomiting are described on pages 110 to 112, and they must be carefully followed to avoid the risk of the serious complication of diabetic ketoacidosis. Because these procedures are so important, they are outlined in the following summary.

If meals are omitted due to loss of appetite or vomiting, you must:

- Never reduce or stop insulin.
- Test the blood. If the blood tests show the blood glucose to be within the normal range, continue with the normal dose of insulin.
- If the blood glucose is very high, increase the dose of insulin by the amounts recommended by your doctor. Therefore, it is essential that you check these amounts with your doctor before your child is sick.
- Replace meals and snacks by hourly drinks containing sugar, at the rate of one good-sized glassful every hour. These drinks can be fruit juices, Lucozade, or other sweetened drinks, such as ordinary Coca-Cola or lemonade.
- Continue to test the blood, and give sweetened drinks until your child is eating normally again.
- If your doctor considers it necessary, give an additional dose of short-acting insulin.
- Vomiting, nausea or loss of appetite usually lasts only a relatively short time, so if your child fails to improve within a few hours, consult your doctor or diabetic clinic.
- Should episodes recur it may be helpful to use tests for ketones (see page 111).

Diabetes and your other children

Inheritance

If you have other children, or you intend having more in the future, you might well be concerned that they, too, could develop diabetes. The risk of Type 1 diabetes being inherited is small (see page 145). In fact, the type of diabetes most commonly inherited is Type 2 diabetes. On the whole, it is recommended that you should plan the family you want and not be put off by the fear of another child having diabetes.

Should my other children be regularly tested?

If you are concerned that your other children might also develop diabetes, you might feel that they should have regular tests to determine whether this is likely to be the case. Unfortunately there is no accurate test at the moment that can predict whether or not somebody is going to develop diabetes. Routine screening, therefore, is not recommended. The best approach is to perform a blood test to put your mind at rest, if at any time you feel that one of your other children shows symptoms of diabetes. If you are uncertain about this ask your doctor to help.

Reactions of your other children to your child with diabetes

A problem often encountered is that a child with diabetes may be seen by their brothers or sisters to be receiving more attention than themselves. This may lead to misunderstandings and it is wise, therefore, to remind your other children of the disadvantages and difficulties of having diabetes.

A topic which you must discuss with your other children is the problem of hypoglycaemia and how to deal with it. They should be taught to give sugar during a reaction, and to make sure that an adult is told. Severe hypoglycaemic reactions, especially if associated with a fit, can be very alarming to a small brother or sister, but if they are forewarned then they may not be so frightened.

Diabetes and the family diet

Many parents are surprised to learn that the diet for diabetes is the same healthy diet recommended for everyone. Such a diet contains very little sugar, which damages the teeth, and sufficient carbohydrate, protein and fat to ensure full growth and development, but not

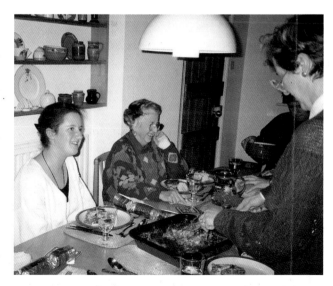

so much that it causes obesity. Your family may react strongly at first to any reduction in sweet food and drinks, but it is surprising how quickly children, in particular, can develop a taste for savoury food. Older members of the family, with long-established eating habits, will probably be the most resistant to change, even though they may appreciate the possible benefits of a healthier diet.

Finally, despite the difficulties you may encounter, the vast majority of children with diabetes grow up in the normal way and live healthy, long and productive lives.

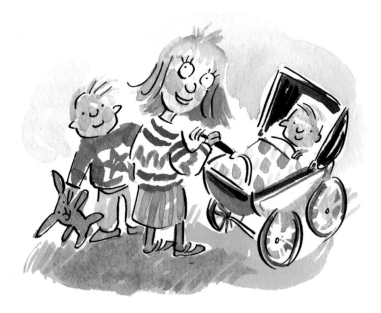

11 Diabetes and Your Daily Life

One of the main aims of your treatment is that diabetes should interfere as little as possible with your day-to-day activities. In general your treatment should be adapted to allow you to carry on as near normally as possible. However, some modifications may be necessary. This chapter describes areas in your daily life that may concern you.

■ Will it affect my work?

The vast majority of people taking insulin are able to continue or to take up work in the normal way. You should be able to function as well as – if not better than – you did before you developed diabetes.

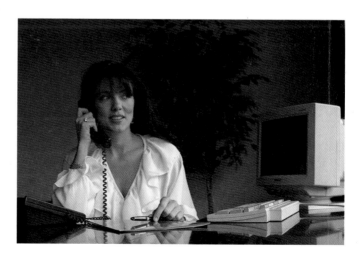

Almost all types of occupation are open to people taking insulin. However, there are some restrictions for those jobs where the development of hypoglycaemia could put other people at risk.

■ You are not allowed to fly aeroplanes, hold a public service driving licence or drive heavy goods vehicles and may be restricted from driving any vehicles over 3.5 tonnes (Group 2). These restrictions have been imposed to safeguard other people, since if you were to have a hypoglycaemic reaction your vehicle could go out of control.

■ The Armed Services, the Police Force and the Fire Service all require strict standards of health. Whereas you might be perfectly all right if you have a hypoglycaemic reaction, other people's safety could be jeopardised. Consequently these services do not generally accept those with Type 1 diabetes. If, however, you develop diabetes while in service, arrangements can usually be made to keep you in employment.

■ Restrictions are also imposed on those working on ships since they may be away from adequate medical help for long periods of time.

■ If you have a potentially dangerous occupation, such as deep-sea diving or steeplejacking, you will probably have to change your job. If you never have reactions you may think such a step is unnecessary. However, simply ask yourself: 'If I should have a reaction when doing my job, could I harm myself or cause injury to other people?' If the answer is 'Yes', then perhaps you should consider an alternative career.

Applying for a job

It is often felt that employers might discriminate against people with diabetes. When this occurs, it is usually because the employer is misinformed or unaware of the true facts about diabetes. Usually, however, if you are the best applicant, you will get the job. If you should find that your explanations are not being accepted, then you should consider asking your doctor to talk to your would-be employer. Alternatively, you could ask your doctor to provide a reference prior to making your job application. When employers appreciate the self-discipline you require to control your diabetes, then they may consider you to be a rather better bet than other applicants. This is confirmed by the above-average work record of most people with diabetes. You may be tempted to conceal the fact that you have diabetes – don't, it may only cause problems later, especially if you have an unexpected hypoglycaemic reaction.

How diabetes affects your job

To carry out your job effectively you will need to keep your diabetes well controlled. It will be necessary for you to have regular breaks for snacks, and to have your meals on time. This should be explained to your employer, together with the fact that you could suffer a hypoglycaemic reaction. You should, however, reassure your employer, by stressing that:

- Most hypoglycaemic attacks are prevented by eating regularly. Usually they are very short-lived, and are easily relieved within a minute or so by taking sugar or its equivalent.
- Severe attacks involving loss of consciousness are extremely rare.
- The dangers to which you might be exposed when working with machinery are minimal, and the warning symptoms of hypoglycaemia will prevent major incidents.

You must ensure that you do not let your blood glucose go too low when in charge of a vehicle. Driving a car or other Group 1 vehicle (but not a Group 2 vehicle) should be no problem (see pages 204 to 207).

It is also important that your work colleagues know that you have diabetes. If, for example, they detect symptoms of hypoglycaemia before you do, then they can alert you; it will also prove very useful if they know exactly what to do if you should have an exceptionally bad attack.

What about shifts?

Do not be put off taking work which involves extended hours, shift working, etc. It is always possible to work out a system of insulin injections to match your work and meal times. Use of the pen system of injection with small injections of fast-acting insulin will enable you to switch from night to day shifts or to work on jobs that require variable working hours.

Starting work for the first time

You may have discovered that you needed less insulin when at school than when you were on holiday. Likewise, when working, especially if your job involves manual labour, you will probably need to reduce your insulin. It is a wise precaution, therefore, to reduce your insulin slightly on the day you start work. Take some tests and, if the glucose level is low, have extra carbohydrate.

It is essential that you continue to take your snacks or meals at the correct times. You may feel embarrassed to ask for breaks when your colleagues continue working. It is much more embarrassing to have a hypoglycaemic reaction. Always choose food which is small and easily chewed and swallowed.

When you start work for the first time you may find that your injection and breakfast times will have to be earlier than when you were at school. If that is the case, you should bring forward the time of your snack.

■ Financial considerations

Insurance

On all insurance proposals where data are required for underwriting assessment, it is imperative that statements are made in good faith. There must be full disclosure of material facts. If it transpires that there has been non-disclosure of any material fact, then the contract can be repudiated. On most proposals, specific questions are asked to elicit certain information, and for many types of insurance, diabetes is a fact which underwriters will wish to consider. Disclosure will enable the insurer to ask for supplementary information, to seek a report from your doctor, or to ask for a medical examination if it is considered necessary.

Diabetes UK provides its own full range of insurance services. You can read more about this in Chapter 12 (page 216).

Life assurance

Because of the possibility of long-term complications, it is usual for some premium loading to be placed on life assurance. The loading applied to term assurance, such as mortgage protection, is likely to be higher than that applied to whole life or endowment policies.

Motor insurance

You are advised in the section on driving (page 207) of the need for full and honest statements to insurance companies. Your insurer may ask for an additional premium, although many companies will quote normal rates, provided you have not been involved in an accident attributable to your diabetes.

Permanent sickness and accident insurance

For this type of insurance you are likely to have to pay higher than normal premiums.

Travel and personal accident insurance

This is a field of insurance in which you need to be especially careful. If you take out such a policy, you should pay particular attention to the exclusion clauses, which normally exclude all pre-existing illness.

Pensions/superannuation

You should not encounter any problems negotiating normal pension and superannuation rights.

Other financial considerations

- Prescription charges in the UK are waived for all people taking insulin. A form (FP92A) will be signed by your doctor, which will enable you to obtain an exemption certificate. This applies to all prescriptions, whether related to your diabetes or not.
- Travel to hospital clinics, if frequent, may be a financial problem. Again, help can often be obtained by discussion with your doctor or hospital social worker.
- Those who develop late complications, especially with their eyes, may be eligible for additional benefits.

Sport and outdoor activities

What can you or can't you do?

There are very few sports in which those with insulin-treated diabetes have not competed or indeed excelled. Athletics of all kinds, first-class professional football, mountaineering, marathon running and the usual activities of a less tiring type, such as gardening and walking, are all within the capabilities of people on insulin.

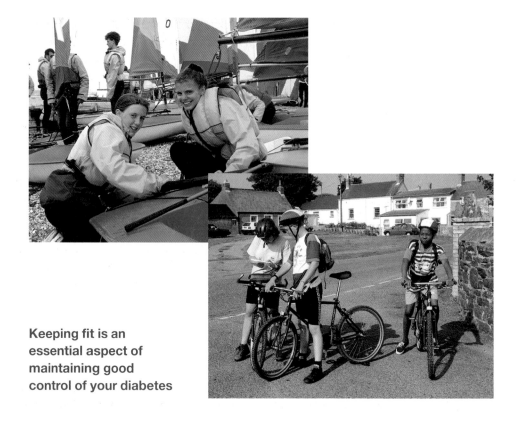

Keeping fit is an essential aspect of maintaining good control of your diabetes

With one or two exceptions, you should not give up sporting activities. Indeed, good physical fitness will help your diabetes control by making the action of insulin on your fat and muscle cells more efficient. It will also help prevent later problems with your circulation.

However, strenuous activities such as swimming, football or heavy manual work use up glucose. Unless you have more carbohydrate or reduce your insulin dose you will run the risk of a hypoglycaemic reaction.

For relatively unplanned exercise, such as suddenly deciding to play squash, go for a jog or dig the garden, it is better to increase your carbohydrate intake than to change your insulin dose. The amount of extra carbohydrate needed varies from person to person. It is also influenced by the strenuousness of the activity. You should certainly allow extra carbohydrate for swimming, and more if you are a distance swimmer. Four strips of Kit Kat or a mini Mars bar are quickly absorbed, and should do the trick for exercise lasting for thirty minutes to an hour. For ball games such as football, make sure you have some extra carbohydrate at half-time. As you will probably be thirsty, it is easy to take extra carbohydrate in the form of a drink such as fruit juice or Lucozade. Carry some glucose sweets or Dextrosol in your pocket for emergencies.

If, however, you have regular or planned sessions, such as Saturday afternoon football, training sessions, booked times in a fitness centre, or PE classes, a reduction in insulin dosage is sensible. You will usually also need to eat some extra carbohydrate, but not as much as if you didn't reduce your insulin.

Remember that the effect of exercise may not occur for several hours after you have stopped. This is especially so after hard training sessions or prolonged exercise.

If you take all the necessary precautions, strenuous activities should not cause any problems. For example, if you should have a hypo while playing football, no great harm will result. Simply sit down, have some glucose, and play again when you feel better.

Where caution is necessary

There are two types of sport where you need to exercise special care: those which may be termed 'risky' sports, and those where you might drive yourself to exhaustion. 'Risky' sports – swimming, sub-aqua diving, hang gliding, solo sailing or mountaineering – are clearly not advisable if you are prone to hypoglycaemia. You would not be able to eat a lump of sugar while hanging below a glider and therefore might lapse into unconsciousness! As with work, you should always ask yourself: 'If I develop hypoglycaemia while doing X, could I take my sugar? If not, would I be in danger and would I put anybody else at risk?'

In all high-risk activities you need to take extra precautions. They may seem obvious enough, but in the excitement of the moment they are easily forgotten. Taking rock climbing and mountaineering as examples, here is what you should do:

■ Measure your blood glucose before setting off.

■ Take emergency supplies of insulin and glucose.

■ Take enough food for twice as long as you think you will be away, and also take into account the extra activity you will be doing.

■ Since there will be other people with you, split the emergency supplies between you, so that if your rucksack drops off the rock face, all is not lost.

Swimming is another potentially risky sport, and you should always follow these simple rules:

■ Never go swimming alone.

■ Whoever accompanies you must know how to treat a hypo and have the means to do so.

■ Never go swimming at times when hypoglycaemia is most likely to occur – just before a meal, for example.

■ Have a 'swimming snack' before you start.

Thus, the message is simple: hypoglycaemic reactions are unpleasant and should be prevented if at all possible. They are dangerous only if they occur in a potentially dangerous situation, such as when in a swimming bath.

Sports which can lead to exhaustion, such as marathon running and professional sports, are not prohibited, but special care is necessary to avoid getting very short of fuel or liquid. First, you must get trained. Build up your distances slowly. While you are doing this you should test the effect of reducing your insulin before your training session. Test your blood before and after. You must not get short of fluid. You need to have a combination of longer-acting carbohydrate, eg sandwiches or digestive biscuits, together with some instant energy before you start. The instant energy is best taken in the form of slightly salted and sugary drink. You need to top these up every couple of miles. When the race is over replace any fluid you have lost with more glucose or fluid. Once you have recovered have some more longer-acting carbohydrate. You will then avoid the delayed effects which may cause hypoglycaemia.

Exercise and high blood sugars

Although the usual effect of exercise is to lower the blood sugar, occasionally the reverse occurs. This happens if you have too little insulin – the glucose cannot be used by the exercising muscles and blood glucose rises. This does not usually matter unless the exercise is very strenuous (as above – marathon racing, professional sports and intensive training regimens).

Therefore, if you feel unwell, ie cold/sore throat, etc, and your blood sugar is on the high side, avoid very strenuous exercise, or delay until the glucose level is lower, and certainly do not reduce your insulin.

■ Travel, holidays and diabetes

You should be able to travel on holiday or business, either in this country or abroad, in exactly the same way as anybody else.

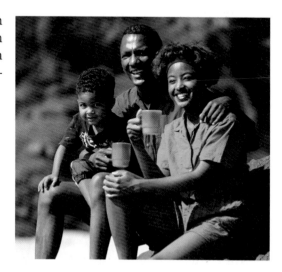

Who should know that you have diabetes?

If you are not travelling with your family, it is sensible to let any travelling companions know that you have diabetes. They should know where you keep your glucose, and be aware of the need to seek medical help in an emergency. It could also be helpful if they know how to give an injection of insulin if, say, you were to injure your arm in a skiing accident, or an injection of glucagon (see page 118).

When travelling by air, it is wise to let members of the cabin crew know that you have diabetes.

Identification

In case of language difficulties, always carry your diabetic identity card, and preferably one translated into the language of the country you are visiting.

Vaccinations

You can receive all necessary vaccinations in the same way as someone without diabetes.

Travel sickness

You should always remind yourself when planning a journey that even though travel is commonplace, journeys are not always smooth.

If you are prone to travel sickness you should ask your doctor for tablets beforehand. Kwells are mild but safe, whereas antihistamines are stronger but may make you drowsy. Take some sweetened fruit juices, which you may need to drink if you are unable to eat your usual meals. You should also take the usual steps to increase your insulin if your tests indicate an increase in blood glucose.

Your insulin and syringe

You should always carry your insulin and syringe/pen with you in your hand luggage. This is allowed by airlines, and you should always refuse to give them to anyone (even if they promise to give them to the cabin staff for safe-keeping until you need them).

Never carry insulin and other supplies in your main baggage if this is to be placed in the hold of an aeroplane. The insulin will freeze, affecting its potency.

To avoid any problems, particularly with Customs or police, you should always have some formal means of identifying yourself as having diabetes. A Diabetes UK card, Medicalert, SOS bracelet or necklace or a letter from the clinic will ensure problems are avoided.

Insulin availability

Insulin is available in all developed countries and in most others as well, at least in the main cities. However, the type, strength and purity may differ from your usual insulin, so it is best to take adequate amounts with you. If, however, you are going to reside abroad for, say, one or two years, you should enquire beforehand about the availability of supplies locally. Your NHS family doctor is not allowed to give you a bulk supply of insulin if you intend to reside abroad for some months. He can, however, give you enough to see you through any reasonable holiday period.

Insulin will remain fully active for at least one month at a temperature of 25°C (77°F). Thus, it is only in very hot climates that you will need to be more careful. Keeping the insulin in a water container in your bathroom usually suffices. If you are staying for more than a couple of weeks, arrange to keep your spare insulin in a refrigerator.

However, insulin stored in the glove compartment or on the dashboard or rear window ledge of a car left in full sunshine will rapidly deteriorate, not only in Mediterranean countries, but even in Scotland! In tropical countries keep your insulin in a pre-cooled vacuum flask when travelling.

Dehydration

If you visit countries with tropical or very hot climates you will sweat more than when at home. This may cause a significant loss of salt and water. If severe this will cause sunstroke (more correctly called heat stroke). This is a hazard for everyone newly arrived in the tropics, but with diabetes could lead to a serious loss of fluid. Therefore, it is important to take a few simple precautions.

- Maintain an adequate intake of water and salt.
- Do not over-exert yourself until you are acclimatised.
- Wear loose-fitting and comfortable clothing, including a hat.
- Keep your body covered and avoid sunburn.

Sickness

One of the commonest problems among travellers is diarrhoea. Very rarely, it may be due to a serious infection, such as typhoid or paratyphoid fever, or cholera. Vaccination offers some protection against these. In addition, it is essential to take adequate hygiene and preventive measures. These will also be of some help against the less serious, but still troublesome and very much more common, 'traveller's tummy':

- Do not drink unbottled water unless you boil it or add sterilising tablets.

- Avoid uncooked foods and vegetables and fruit you have not peeled.
- If you eat shellfish, make sure they are fresh and well cooked.
- Avoid all foods that have been cooked and then cooled, such as cold buffets and puddings.
- Obtain some antibiotic tablets from your doctor before leaving, and take these according to his/her instructions.

In the case of illness, you should follow your usual precautions and if necessary increase your insulin. Never reduce it. Fortunately, most tummy upsets are of short duration, and are nearly always due to a change in diet, so that with care you should be able to manage without medical help.

Availability of medical assistance

This is rarely free. Countries in the EU have reciprocal medical cover. Before you go you must fill in a Form E111, available from your local DSS office or Post Office, in order to get the necessary certificate to prove you are eligible for the treatment. Even then, the cover may not be as comprehensive as in this country. Thus, it is essential, especially where no reciprocal arrangement exists, to take out adequate medical insurance. Check the small print of any travel policy carefully, as 'pre-existing' conditions, such as diabetes, may well not be covered. If you should experience any difficulty in obtaining this type of insurance, Diabetes UK Insurance Services can help you (see Chapter 12, page 216).

Finally, always carry a card indicating that you have diabetes requiring insulin treatment (see page 117).

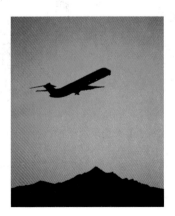

Air travel

People taking insulin often worry that air travel is going to impose difficulties. However, it is all much simpler than it would first appear. You should not be discouraged from going wherever you want to. With some simple adjustments you will be able to keep control of your diabetes. One of the major concerns is that you might go hypoglycaemic. However, with the excitement of travel and the frequent meals served on planes people are more likely to go high than low.

Short flights (less than about five hours)

These pose no problems at all. The time difference between your departure point and destination is likely to be no more than an hour or two. Just carry on as normal, having your insulin at the normal times. Remember, however, that if you are leaving late morning you may not get a meal for an hour or so into the flight. Sometimes planes are delayed. Always carry some snacks with you, either in the form of digestive biscuits or some extra sandwiches, so that if a meal time is delayed you can have something to eat and avoid going low.

Always carry your insulin syringes or pen and a good supply of insulin and testing equipment with you. Luggage can go astray.

Long-haul flights

These are a bit more complicated. You will be crossing time zones which may seem confusing. Let's look at some examples.

Going east

London to Singapore

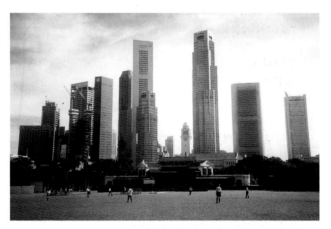

Assume that a flight leaves at 10 pm (2200 hrs). You will have to check in at about 8 pm (2000 hrs). The flight time is about 11 hours. You will be given two meals, one served two to three hours after you have taken off and one about two hours before you land. You can get a snack between times if you need it. You would arrive at about 9 am (0900 hrs) British time or 5 pm (1700 hrs) local time.

The best thing would be to:

- Have maybe half the dose of the insulin you normally have before your evening meal at around 5 to 6 pm (1700 to 1800 hrs) before you set off for the flight.
- Follow this by a snack, then take the other half of the insulin just before the evening meal served on the flight.

Another meal will be served two hours or so before you land. If you are asleep you will usually be woken with a fruit juice or freshening towel just before this. Have another injection just before this meal, perhaps similar to your normal pre-breakfast dose. This will be at about 7 am (0700 hrs) British time but 3 pm (1500 hrs) local time!

After disembarking and getting to your hotel it will probably be about 6 or 7 pm (1800 or 1900 hrs). You can then go back to your normal evening dose followed by a meal and going to bed.

Singapore to Perth

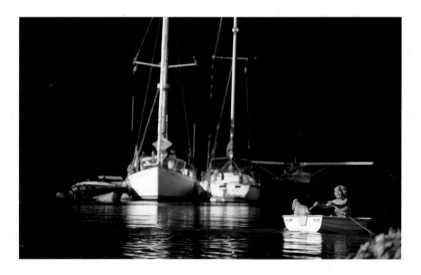

After landing in Singapore there will probably be a two hour delay before taking off again (which will be about 7 pm (1900 hrs) Singapore time). A meal will be served a couple of hours after that, so take another dose of insulin (say half your normal pre-evening meal dose) before the main meal is served on the flight. You would then arrive in Perth five hours after departure from Singapore at about 1 am (0100 hrs) Perth time. By the time you have disembarked, collected your luggage and settled into your hotel it will be about 3 am (0300 hrs) – have a snack preceded by the other half of your normal evening dose. Go to bed and start again as usual at 8 or 9 am (0800 or 0900 hrs).

British Time	Singapore Time			Meals	Suggested time of insulin injection
1700				Snack	Half normal pre-evening meal dose
2000			Check-in		
2200			Flight departs London		
2400				Meal	Other half normal pre-evening meal dose
0700	1500			Breakfast	Normal morning insulin
0900	1700		Flight arrives Singapore		
1100	1900		Arrive hotel	Meal	Normal evening meal meal insulin
British Time	**Singapore Time**	**Perth Time**		**Meals**	**Suggested time of insulin injection**
1100	1900	2000	Flight departs Singapore		
1300	2100	2200		Meal	Half normal pre-evening meal dose
1600	2400	0100	Flight arrives Perth		
		0300	Arrive hotel	Have a snack	Other half normal pre-evening meal dose

Going west

London to New York

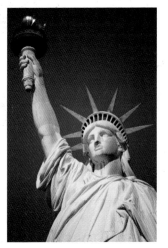

Assume that you are leaving London at 11 am (1100 hrs). You should have your normal pre-breakfast insulin and breakfast.

Have a small snack just before you get on the plane. A meal will be served two to three hours into the flight. That will be at about 1 to 2 pm (1300 to 1400 hrs) British time. If you are used to taking three or four injections a day have a small injection of insulin as usual before the 'lunch' meal.

Another snack will be served just before you land, which will be at about 5.30 pm (1730 hrs) British time. It is better not to have insulin before this snack. Your arrival time will be at about 7 pm (1900 hrs) British time or 2 pm (1400 hrs) US time. Once you are off the aircraft and have arrived at your hotel have a snack and settle in. You will probably have another meal around 6 pm (1800 hrs), and should take your normal pre-evening meal insulin. Get back to normal the next day.

British Time	New York Time		Meals	Suggested time of insulin injection
0800			Breakfast	Normal morning dose
0900		Check-in		
			Snack	
1100		Flight departs London		
1300			Meal	Normal lunchtime dose (if you usually take this)
1730			Snack*	
1900				
	1400	Flight arrives New York		
	1600	Arrive hotel	Snack	
	1800		Meal	Normal pre-evening meal dose
	2200		Snack	Bedtime dose (if taken)

* You should have some biscuits with you to take earlier if you feel the need.

London to San Francisco

The flight is eleven hours long, so if you depart at 11 am (1100 hrs) you would arrive at 10 pm (2200 hrs) British time. Two meals would be served, the first two to three hours into the flight and the second two hours before landing.

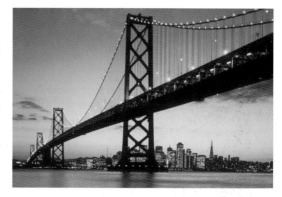

Take your morning insulin as usual, have a snack before getting on to the plane and, if you take insulin before your lunch, do this just before the meal is served on the plane.

The next meal will be served on the plane at about 7 to 8 pm (1900 to 2000 hrs) British time, so have the equivalent of half your normal pre-evening meal dose of insulin just before this. If you usually take a mixture of quick- and slow-acting insulin in the evening, only take the quick-acting.

You will disembark at around 2 pm (1400 hrs) US time. When you get to your hotel at about 5 or 6 pm (1700 or 1800 hrs), have your normal pre-evening meal insulin before your evening meal, and get back to normal the next morning.

Jet lag

Jet lag may cause you to wake at unusual times in the early hours of the morning for the first night or two. Try to avoid starting the day too early. If you are wide awake just have a little snack and try to go back to sleep until your normal getting up time, when you can restart your normal morning insulin.

Hints

It is also a good idea to have drinks of mineral water or unsweetened juice every hour or so. You can get very dry in the atmosphere of an aircraft, and if you have plenty to drink you will feel generally fresher and better when the flight ends.

Giving insulin injections on the flight is actually quite easy to do without going to the toilet. You can inject either into your abdomen or the back of your calves or upper arm. It is sensible to wear loose fitting clothing so that you can get access to the injection site without too much commotion.

Finally, be careful with alcohol. Generally speaking, on long-distance flights drinking a lot of alcohol can make you feel pretty rough, and it certainly complicates matters if you are taking insulin as well.

If all this seems too confusing, discuss your planned trip with your doctor or specialist nurse. For people on multiple injections these adjustments are very easy. They are slightly more difficult when taking fixed mixtures, and you may wish to ask for some quick-acting insulin just to use on the flight. Your specialist nurse should be able to advise you about this.

■ Emigration

Uncomplicated diabetes should be no bar to emigration. A certificate of health is normally required, and you will need a statement from your doctor to say that your diabetes is reasonably well controlled. There may be more problems if you suffer from any complications, but this will need to be discussed with the emigration department concerned or your own doctor. In either case, remember that healthcare in the country you are going to may not be free, and you should, therefore, take out the appropriate health insurance cover. You should also take a letter from your doctor, containing details of your treatment. Remember, too, that some countries may not be using U100 insulin, in which case you will require a change of insulin strength and syringe.

■ Social life

Evening parties, discos and dances

If you are to enjoy an active social life the time of your evening meal may need to be altered. So, what do you do if you are invited to a party at which the meal is planned for, say, 8 pm, when you normally have your evening injection at 5.30 pm and your meal at 6.00 pm?

The answer is straightforward:

- Delay your injection until 7.30 pm.
- Have a snack, eg a sandwich, at your normal evening meal time (fruit juice is quick-acting and will not spoil your appetite).
- Assume the meal will be late; be prepared to have an extra snack if the meal is very late.
- If you are used to taking regular quick-acting insulin before each meal, take half the dose of your usual evening injection before your snack and the remainder when you have your proper meal.

If you have only one injection a day, 'reverse' the evening meal and bedtime snack, so that you have a snack at, say, 6 pm, to tide you over until the meal at 8 pm.

When you go to a party or disco:

- Try to have your evening injection and meal at the usual time.
- If the party or disco starts early, and food and drink are available, have a small evening meal. Take a snack with you and eat either this or food from the buffet two to three hours later.
- Disco type parties may include a lot of exercise. It is possibly wise to reduce your evening quick-acting insulin by a couple of units. Top it up with snacks if the party is prolonged.
- Watch the alcohol – this can cause hypoglycaemia (see Chapters 3 and 10).

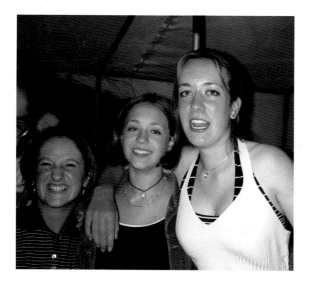

Don't let your diabetes put you off dancing – enjoy yourself! But remember, dancing is exercise and you may need more to eat and drink

■ Driving

Points to remember

You must:

- ■ Tell your insurance company that you have diabetes.
- ■ Tell the licensing authorities (DVLA, Swansea, SA99 1AT) that you have diabetes.

Filling in the licence application form (D1)

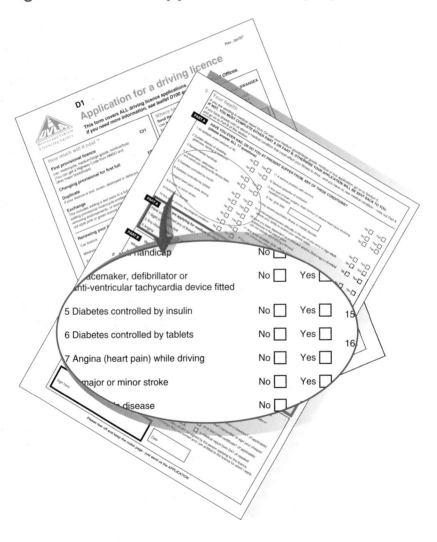

When you apply for a driving licence you have to answer one question of particular importance to you. Question 5A asks:

■ 5A.   Have you ever had, or do you at present suffer from any of these conditions:

You must tick the 'yes' box for 'Diabetes controlled by insulin'.

For Question 5B 'What is the condition?', write in the box 'Insulin Treated Diabetes'. For the question 'Has it got worse since you told us about it?' you can usually tick the 'no' box.

After you have completed and returned your application form, you may be sent a supplementary form, asking for further information, including the name and address of your doctor or hospital clinic, as well as your consent to allow the Driver and Vehicle Licensing Authority to approach your doctor directly. This procedure does not mean that you will be refused a driving licence.

Provided that you demonstrate satisfactory control, recognise your low blood glucose level symptoms and have satisfactory eyesight, ordinary driving licences for all vehicles in Group 1 will be granted to you. These include all motor cycles and cars, and lorries up to 3.5 tonnes. The licence will normally be issued for three years and renewals will be made free of charge.

If your diabetes has been diagnosed only recently and you hold a 'life' licence, this will be revoked and replaced with a 'period' licence. Renewals can take several weeks, but should your licence pass its expiry date you can continue to drive, providing you have made application for a renewal.

Insurance cover

It is compulsory by law for every driver to be insured against the risk of liability for injury to third parties. Most insurers are willing to offer insurance cover to those with diabetes at standard rates, but some may wish to charge a higher premium. Some insurers will require a medical report from your doctor, who is entitled to charge a fee for this service. If you have difficulty with insurance, Diabetes UK can help and advise you.

You must tell your insurers that you have diabetes, no matter how questions on the insurance proposal form may be phrased. Upon diagnosis, existing policy holders must immediately advise their insurers. If you withhold this information and are then involved in an accident, the insurers could be entitled to repudiate your claim, by making the policy null and void on the grounds of non-disclosure.

When not to drive

You should not drive if:

- You are being started on insulin; you should wait until stabilisation is complete.
- You have difficulty in recognising early symptoms of hypoglycaemia.
- You have any problems with your eyesight that cannot be corrected by glasses.

Driving heavy goods vehicles, minibuses and public service vehicles

If you need insulin treatment you are generally restricted from driving large lorries or buses – Group 2 vehicles. These include all lorries greater than 3.5 tonnes. Driving minibuses with fewer than nine seats is allowed, but not larger ones. Exemptions may exist for those driving minibuses for charitable purposes or for those who drive larger vehicles as part of their job. Stricter medical requirements will apply. This should be discussed with the DVLA. You are also unable to hold a passenger vehicle licence.

Alcohol

Never drink and drive. If you are on insulin, a hypoglycaemic reaction may look like drunkenness; if your breath smells of alcohol, suspicions will be heightened. Furthermore, it should be borne in mind that heavy drinking, particularly of spirits, may provoke hypoglycaemia.

Hypoglycaemia and driving

The dangers of hypoglycaemia while driving are obvious and you must make sure it never happens. Therefore, never drive for more than two hours without a break for a snack.

As soon as you experience any warning signs:

- Stop the car
- Turn off the ignition
- Leave the driving seat until fully recovered
- Have something to eat: always keep a supply of biscuits and glucose in the car.

If you are found to be hypoglycaemic when in charge of a motor vehicle, especially if you are involved in an accident, you lose your licence for a minimum of six months. This is a very good reason for keeping your diabetes well controlled. Many people find blood testing invaluable as a means of checking that they are safe to drive, without always taking excess carbohydrate 'just in case'.

There can never be any excuse for a reaction while driving: it can never be due to bad luck, only to bad management.

■ Diabetes and smoking

The dangers of smoking are well known.

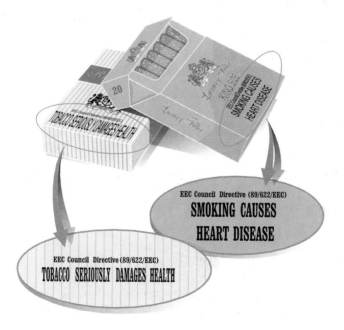

If you want to avoid these risks, DON'T SMOKE.

■ Diabetes and drugs

It is illegal to possess drugs, such as marijuana, pot, speed, etc. Even so, you may know people who have smoked pot or taken pep pills without coming to any apparent harm. However, for you to take drugs which alter the way your brain works would be dangerous and could possibly be fatal. One of the most serious effects of such drugs is that they cause you to lose your awareness of the warning signs of hypoglycaemia, and at a party where drugs are available it is unlikely that anyone would notice (or care) if you became severely hypoglycaemic. Ecstasy, especially taken under 'rave' circumstances, may be particularly dangerous. The dehydration associated with prolonged dancing has caused diabetic ketoacidosis, coma, or even death. Topping up with fluids may not prevent this. Often insulin injections or adequate carbohydrate intake may be overlooked after taking drugs. Do not take unnecessary risks by taking drugs that have not been prescribed for you.

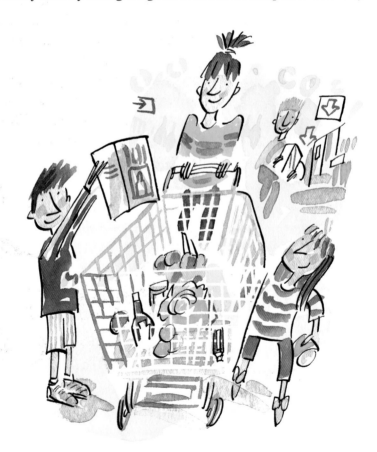

12 Diabetes UK

Being diagnosed with diabetes can leave you feeling very confused and isolated. If you have lots of unanswered questions about your diabetes, need advice on how diabetes might affect your home life or your work, or want to be put in touch with other people with diabetes, contact Diabetes UK. The organisation is here to work with you to improve the level of diabetes care available. It is a medical self-help charity that has both lay and professional members, and has been working with people with diabetes for over 60 years. This chapter describes Diabetes UK's work and invites you to support them.

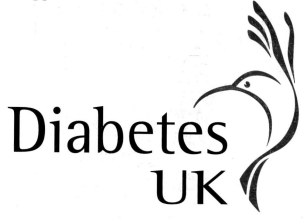

■ Diabetes UK's history

Diabetes UK (the new name for the British Diabetic Association) was founded in 1934 by R D Lawrence, a diabetologist who had diabetes himself, and H G Wells, the author of books such as *The Time Machine* and *War of the Worlds*. The organisation's aims remain the same as they were in the 1930s: to help and care for people with diabetes and those close to them, to represent and campaign for their interests, and to fund research into diabetes. But advances in medical and information technology since the charity was founded mean that today Diabetes UK can pursue these goals in ways that even H G Wells could never have foreseen.

■ Providing care and advice

Diabetes UK Careline

To help you understand and manage your diabetes Diabetes UK runs a careline. Diabetes UK Careline is a confidential service which offers

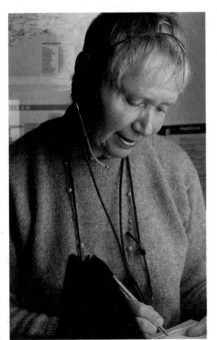

information and support on diabetes by telephone, letter, fax or email. Diabetes UK Careline staff cannot comment on your individual medical situation – your doctor or specialist nurse is in the best position to do this – but they can talk over any difficulties you may be having and send you information on a wide range of diabetes-related subjects.

Diabetes UK Careline staff are trained in diabetes and also have counselling experience. You may wish to talk in confidence about a difficult or distressing situation; you do not have to give your name or address to receive help.

Diabetes UK Careline deals with calls and letters on a wide range of subjects related to diabetes, including hypoglycaemia, complications, employment, driving, schools, holidays, blood glucose testing and many, many more. Sometimes the phone lines are very busy so you may not always get through the first time you try.

Diabetes UK Careline's telephone number is 020 7424 1030, Textphone (for hard of hearing and deaf) 020 7424 1031. The lines are open Monday to Friday, 9 am–5 pm. Careline can also be contacted by email: careline@ diabetes.org.uk.

Care Developments

The Care Developments team supports Diabetes UK Careline staff and provides the organisation with nursing and diabetes expertise.

The team's role is to ensure that Diabetes UK keeps up to date with developments in diabetes and produces information sheets and leaflets for people with diabetes on all aspects of living with the condition.

Care Developments also provides information through *Balance*, Diabetes UK's bimonthly magazine, and through its website, as well as responding to individual enquiries.

Care Interventions

The Care Interventions team works to identify and develop activity and information for people with diabetes at key points in their lives.

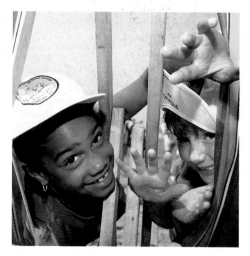

The Youth and Family Events section runs educational holidays and family weekend events for families with a child with diabetes. These annual events offer families an opportunity to meet others and discuss and address ways forward to improve their understanding and management of the condition.

In addition, the Project Development section is continually developing new activities to support people with diabetes at and around the time of diagnosis.

■ Sharing experiences

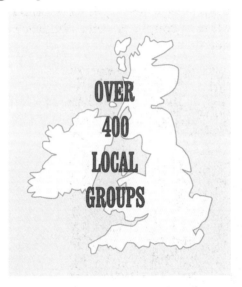

Adjusting to the knowledge that you or a member of your family has diabetes takes time and it is often helpful to meet other people who live with diabetes and have been through a similar situation. They can offer understanding, help and support at an important time. A good way of finding this help is to join a local Diabetes UK voluntary group. There are over 400 across Britain and Northern Ireland, all run voluntarily by people living with diabetes. There are also some specialist groups – for parents and young people with diabetes, South Asian support groups and a group for the visually impaired.

If you would like more information about the groups network, contact Diabetes UK's Voluntary Groups Section. All voluntary groups welcome new members.

Every year, Diabetes UK also organises around 10 *Living with Diabetes* days, which take place on various Saturdays throughout the UK. These take the form of one-day conferences and exhibitions on diabetes, giving you an introduction to life with the condition, how healthcare professionals can help you, and the latest in diabetes research. The conferences are accompanied by exhibitions presented by companies from the pharmaceutical industry who will be promoting their services and products.

■ Spreading the word

Communications are an essential part of Diabetes UK's work. The organisation is uniquely placed to draw together information related to diabetes from the points of view of people with diabetes, carers, healthcare professionals and researchers. As a result, Diabetes UK publishes information which can inform and represent all of these groups, as well as improve the general public's understanding of diabetes.

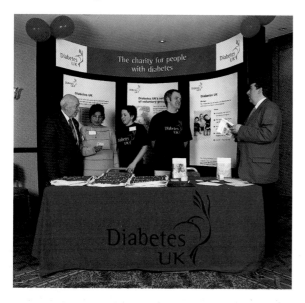

Leaflets and magazines

It is often useful to have your queries backed up with written information, which you can digest later and refer back to. Diabetes UK is the foremost source of leaflets, magazines and books on diabetes – in fact, it has many titles to help you understand more about your condition. Many of the leaflets are free of charge, a number of its publications are available in Welsh and the major Asian languages, and some are available on tape.

In addition to leaflets on single subjects such as *Eating Well, Diabetes and Insurance,* and *The Facts about Insulin,* Diabetes UK also publishes *Balance,* a bimonthly magazine for Diabetes UK members. *Balance* is filled with news, interviews, research updates, recipes and diet information, showing you how you can fit diabetes into an active lifestyle. It is also available on tape and can be bought at larger branches of W H Smith and newsagents. Diabetes UK also publishes a series called *Diabetes for Beginners,* aimed at helping newly diagnosed people.

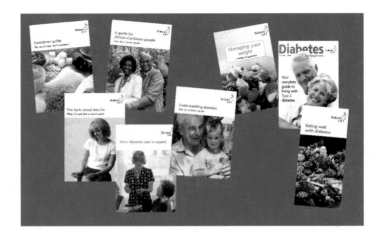

The website

The Internet is a great way both of communicating with other people and of providing information to help you learn more about diabetes. Diabetes UK relaunched its website in June 2000. The site has all the latest news and up-to-date information on diabetes. It covers all areas of diabetes, from *What is diabetes?* and *Managing diabetes*, through to local support and getting involved with Diabetes UK. The online information centre is a particularly useful resource, containing all of Diabetes UK's free publications. There is also a section devoted to research and an area for healthcare professionals. You can find Diabetes UK at http://www.diabetes.org.uk.

Networks for healthcare professionals

Professional conferences

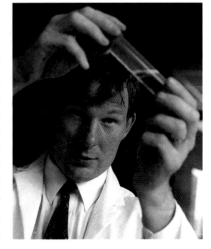

Another important function of Diabetes UK is to spread the news about the latest research and up-to-date guidelines on good diabetes care among the healthcare professionals, eg GPs, nurses, chiropodists and dietitians, who are involved in diabetes care. A number of publications are available to this end, including professional reports setting out recommendations for diabetes care and *Diabetes Update*, a quarterly newsletter for all members of the diabetes care team. There are medical and scientific conferences, held twice a year, which now attract up to 1000 participants. These allow healthcare professionals and scientists to network and give them the opportunity to hear lectures on the latest diabetes research and the various scientific and clinical aspects of the condition.

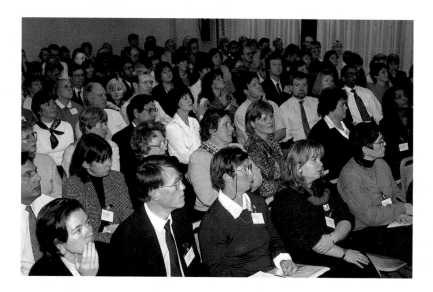

Poster campaigns

Finally, through its poster campaigns Diabetes UK sets out to raise public awareness and funds, and to reach people who may have diabetes but haven't yet been diagnosed. This last is a particularly urgent task given that in the UK alone an estimated one million people are thought to have undetected Type 2 non insulin dependent diabetes. The longer their diabetes goes undetected, the greater their risk of developing complications.

■ Fighting discrimination

Event days and poster campaigns are an important means of raising public awareness of diabetes, and in this way, they are also a key weapon in the fight against discrimination: the more people know about diabetes, the less likely they are to discriminate against people with diabetes. Nevertheless, a good deal of progress still needs to be made in this area, and Diabetes UK is active in opposing discrimination against people with diabetes.

Employment

One major field of discrimination is the job market. Often this sort of discrimination is the result of ignorant outdated ideas about what people with diabetes can and can't do, and may be appealed against under the Disability Discrimination Act. Diabetes UK's Diabetes Care Services can provide you with some of the information you may need to do this.

In some occupations, however, job applicants may come up against an official 'blanket' ban on people with diabetes. Diabetes UK believes that each person with diabetes should be treated as a case in their own right, and has made this argument very successfully in a number of areas of work. It also gives guidance to individuals who find it hard to challenge discrimination. For example, it was decided that firefighters who are diagnosed in service with Type 1 diabetes will no longer be dismissed immediately. Decisions will now be made on a case-by-case basis. Our campaigning work also led to a government review of regulations that originally barred insulin-users from driving vehicles above 3.5 tonnes at work.

Insurance

Another area where people with diabetes have been discriminated against in the past is insurance. Discrimination may come in the form of increased premiums, restricted terms or even cancellation of policies. Diabetes UK Careline used to receive thousands of calls each year from people having problems finding or keeping their driving insurance cover. This situation has been radically improved by the Disability Discrimination Act, but some companies do still charge higher premiums. Revealing that you have diabetes may be problematic, but keeping it a secret from your insurers is even worse. Failure to disclose material facts can invalidate your insurance cover in the event of a claim.

Travel insurance can still be problematic; many travel insurance policies do not include pre-existing medical conditions such as diabetes, so it is important to check carefully before arranging your holiday. As with other policies, the consequences of not mentioning your diabetes may be disastrous, leaving you liable to enormous medical bills.

As far as life assurance policies are concerned, if you already hold a policy when you are diagnosed, you don't need to declare your diabetes. But if you are applying for a new policy you must declare it and expect some loading on your policy.

Faced with the general lack of understanding within the insurance market, Diabetes UK has negotiated its own exclusive schemes to provide policies suited to the needs of people with diabetes and those living with them. Diabetes UK Services offer competitively priced motor and travel insurance, as well as life and home insurance, and other investment products.

■ Leading the way to better care

Through the campaigning activities of Diabetes UK members, considerable improvements in care have been achieved both in hospital clinics and general practice. Over recent years, Diabetes UK has also secured disposable insulin syringes, needles and blood glucose testing strips on NHS prescription. In March 2000, needles and reusable insulin pens also became free to people with diabetes.

Diabetes UK is working closely with the Department of Health on a Diabetes National Service framework, which aims to ensure high standards of care consistently across England. Similar cooperation with government is taking place in Scotland, Wales and Northern Ireland.

Diabetes UK is actively encouraging the development of Local Diabetes Services Advisory Groups (LDSAGs) in local health authorities around the country.

Local Diabetes Services Advisory Groups

An LDSAG is a group of people whose purpose is to be involved in the formation of a local strategy for diabetes services, to advise on and monitor its effects and to recommend the improvements required to provide a service which meets local needs and wishes and national standards. The role and responsibilities of LDSAGs include:

- ■ Developing a local strategy for diabetes care and prevention, with specific objectives and targets.
- ■ Advising on the development of service specification to meet those needs.
- ■ Developing systems to facilitate the achievement of the targets and user satisfaction.
- ■ Monitoring and auditing the quality of the service against the targets and standards set.
- ■ Developing a local information system to assist in this process and identify shortfalls.

Membership includes: representatives of the specialist team and the primary healthcare team, people with diabetes and their carers, commissioners of diabetes services, consultants in public health medicine, managers of provider services, representatives of Diabetes UK voluntary groups and community health centres.

Other members may come from relevant medical specialities, social services, education, health promotion, other voluntary organisations and other relevant local groups or individuals.

Professional membership

Through its professional membership there is close communication between the professionals and Diabetes UK so that its advice and policies are based on and have the support of its professional members. Nearly all doctors specialising in diabetes and specialist nurses, many dietitians and large numbers of general practitioners are members. Primary Care Diabetes UK, one of the professional membership sections, was established to improve co-ordination of care in general practice. The organisation is committed to encouraging high-quality and culturally sensitive primary care for people with diabetes.

The St Vincent Declaration

A significant guide to Diabetes UK's work is the *St Vincent Declaration*, a document compiled in 1989 by diabetes organisations, healthcare professionals and people with diabetes. This sets out targets for reducing the complications of diabetes throughout Europe by improving the way diabetes care is provided.

■ Searching for a cure

Diabetes research is very exciting at the moment, with a number of areas of research at critical stages of development. Diabetes UK is very active in supporting this research. There are usually around 150 Diabetes UK-funded research projects going on throughout the UK, investigating the causes, treatment and prevention of diabetes. Scientists are also looking at hypos, how complications can be prevented, better ways of screening and new targets for treatment design. There are even studies under way looking at some of the psychological aspects of diabetes and what types of diabetes education are most effective.

Diabetes UK is one of the largest funders of diabetes research in the UK. The organisation believes in funding only the highest quality research that promises to make the maximum impact on diabetes. Diabetes UK has two committees: the Research Committee and the Diabetes Development Committee, which between them meet five times each year to decide exactly how money will be spent.

The money for research comes mainly from voluntary sources in the form of donations and legacies. People can ask for their donation to be set aside specifically for the Research Fund or they can support research on a regular basis by joining Diabetes UK Research Focus. Please call Customer Services on 020 7424 1010, or email to customerservice@diabetes.org.uk, for further information.

■ How you can help

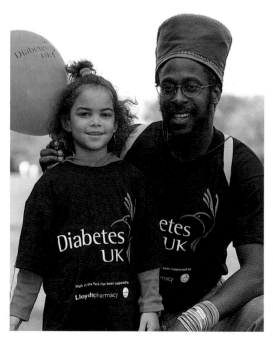

Diabetes UK relies upon its supporters – people with diabetes, their families and friends, and healthcare professionals working in the field – to provide a wide range of services to help people with diabetes. It relies mainly on voluntary donations to fund its research, campaigns and to provide information and support to help people living with diabetes.

If you would like to get involved and help bring about a better future for people with diabetes, please contact the Customer Services team on **020 7424 1010** and they will give you information about:

■ Becoming a member of Diabetes UK
■ Giving regular support to research through Diabetes UK Research Focus
■ Making a donation
■ Holding a fundraising event
■ Giving through your payroll
■ Including Diabetes UK in your will.

If you would like to become involved in any of Diabetes UK's fundraising activities, please get in touch with the Fundraising Department. You may wish to fundraise on your own or with friends, or to be associated with one of Diabetes UK's voluntary groups. The Fundraising Department can point you in whichever direction you prefer.

Your helpful advice and support and your own experiences of living with diabetes are essential to Diabetes UK's work, so do get in touch.

Research Focus

Help to invest in diabetes research – join Diabetes UK Research Focus

Research Focus is Diabetes UK's regular giving scheme dedicated to funding diabetes research. Members of Research Focus each give a regular (monthly, quarterly or annual) amount. This means Research Focus can commit funds to long-term projects, knowing it will have the money to see the project through to its conclusion – a conclusion that it hopes will deliver real benefits for people with diabetes.

Members of Research Focus help fund research into the:

■ Causes of diabetes
■ Genetics of diabetes
■ Secretion and action of insulin
■ Control of diabetes
■ Prevention and treatment of diabetes complications
■ Treatment and care of people with diabetes
■ Psychology of caring for diabetes.

Members of Research Focus give on a regular basis and so provide an ongoing source of funds to invest in diabetes research. Research Focus members who give £5 a month or more receive the annual Research Focus newsletter, an annual review, news items as and when diabetes research developments happen, and invitations to Research Focus Forums where researchers discuss the projects they are working on.

People join Research Focus for a variety of reasons. Some recognise that though a cure for diabetes may be a long way off, it will never be reached if we don't invest in diabetes research now. Others value the potential benefits research may bring to the standard of diabetes care. Many parents with diabetes worry about the genetic link and hope for a day when we can accurately predict if their children will develop diabetes, so we can target future preventative treatments. Whatever the reason, Research Focus members all share the same belief – that research is the key to a better future for people with diabetes. One day, research may even lead us to a cure.

If you share this belief and would like to help achieve it, please contact us for further information about joining Diabetes UK Research Focus.

By letter: Research Focus Manager, Diabetes UK,
              10 Parkway, London NW1 7AA

By phone: 020 7424 1010 (Customer Service Team)
By email: customerservice@diabetes.org.uk

■ How to join Diabetes UK

Diabetes UK is the charity for people with diabetes, working to improve their lives and to achieve our ultimate aim of a future without diabetes – something we could not do or hope for without our members.

Our members help us fund work to:

- ■ Provide **support and information** to people with diabetes so they are informed about their condition and are able to lead a full life.
- ■ **Campaign** for the rights and interests of people with diabetes to ensure they are not discriminated against because of their condition.
- ■ **Provide** answers to the many questions that still surround diabetes and its complications, and make progress towards our ultimate aim of a future without diabetes.

To become a member of Diabetes UK, please contact us for further information.

By letter: Diabetes UK, Customer Services,
              10 Parkway, London NW1 7AA

By phone: 020 7424 1010
By email: customerservice@diabetes.org.uk

What membership of Diabetes UK gives you

- Access to the latest, up-to-date information about diabetes care, research and other issues via our bi-monthly magazine *Balance*, and a wide range of information publications which we produce
- The opportunity to share your experiences with other people with diabetes through our support groups (over 400 nationwide)
- The ability to talk in confidence to Diabetes UK Careline about any diabetes issue or aspect of your diabetes (**020 7424 1030** during office hours)
- A range of insurance and financial products designed specifically with the needs of people with diabetes in mind.

■ National and regional offices

Diabetes UK aims to be closer to its members and to meet their needs as professionally as possible. To this end it has opened regional offices. By having an office in your area it can help ensure the best level of care for people with diabetes and that your voice is heard. Many of Diabetes UK's activities, such as research projects, holidays and network days, are local to your area.

Contact addresses

Diabetes UK
10 Parkway
London
NW1 7AA

Tel: 020 7424 1000
Fax: 020 7424 1001
Email: info@diabetes.org.uk

Diabetes UK Scotland
Savoy House
140 Sauchiehall Street
Glasgow
G2 3HD

Tel: 0141 332 2700
Fax: 0141 332 4880
Email: scotland@diabetes.org.uk

Diabetes UK North West
65 Bewsey Street
Warrington
WA2 7JQ

Tel: 01925 653 281
Fax: 01925 653 288
Email: n.west@diabetes.org.uk

Diabetes UK West Midlands
1 Eldon Court
Eldon Street
Walsall
WS1 2JP

Tel: 01922 614 500
Fax: 01922 646 789
Email: w.midlands@diabetes.org.uk

Diabetes UK Northern Ireland
John Gibson House
257 Lisburn Road
Belfast
BT9 7EN

Tel: 028 9066 6646
Fax: 028 9066 6333
Email: n.ireland@diabetes.org.uk

Diabetes UK Cymru
Quebec House
Castlebridge
Lowbridge Road East
Cardiff
CF11 9AB

Tel:01222 668 276
Fax: 01222 668 329
Email: wales@diabetes.org.uk

Diabetes UK Services

Diabetes UK Services is proud to offer a wide range of highly competitive insurance products that have been developed, in partnership with leading insurance broker Heath Lambert, specifically for people living with diabetes.

As a broker, Heath Lambert can negotiate directly with a range of insurers specifically on issues surrounding diabetes, meaning great deals on travel, motor and home insurance, and financial services.

For the first time, many people who would have previously been excluded will have access to some form of Critical Illness cover on a stand-alone basis.

All services can be reached through the one phone number with a dedicated team of professionals on the other end who understand the issues associated with diabetes.

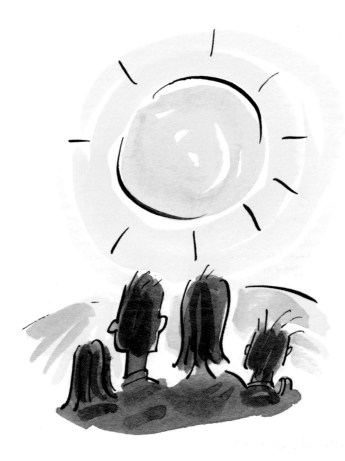

Index

Index compiled by Annette Musker